Where else ca1 0 *of them named,
packed into 100 square miles of mountain scenery? Although
Desolation Wilderness occupies only ⅓ of the area covered by
this guidebook's map, it accounts for ⅚ of its lakes.*

DATE DUE

*The trail makes a brief, steep climb, then winds south to
where ducks mark a 200-yard traverse west to a lodgepole-
shaded camp, perched on a bench above the Rubicon. By it
the river cascades into a 10-foot-deep pool—brisk, but
excellent for diving, cooling off, or just frolicking.*

(Loon Lake Trail)

*The several meadows along this trail will reward wildflower
lovers, while at least three sets of creek pools will please
others. However, the main attractions are the two subalpine
lakes, which by early August can be suitable for swimming.*

(Lyons Creek

D0957828

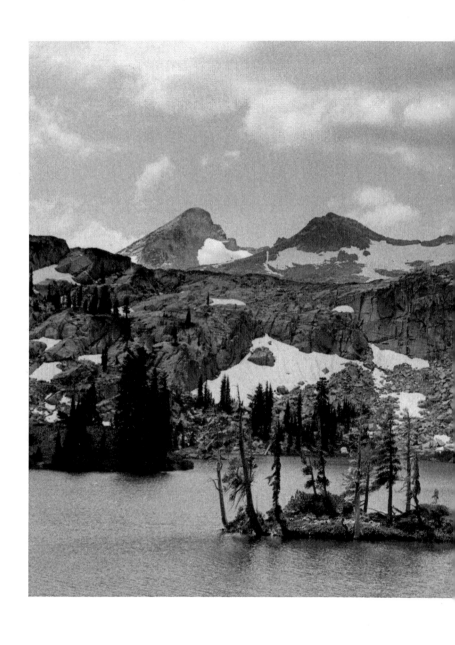

Desolation
Wilderness

and the South Lake Tahoe Basin

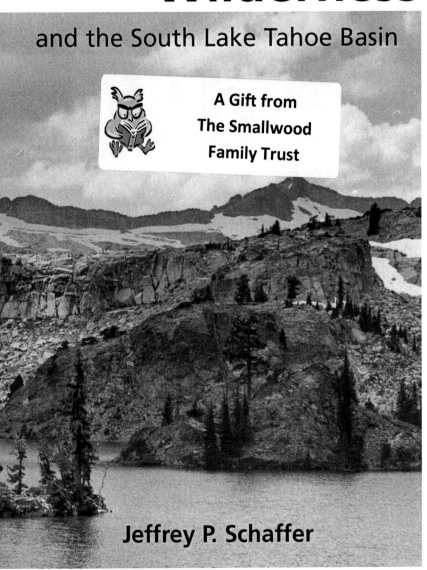

Jeffrey P. Schaffer

WILDERNESS PRESS · BERKELEY, CA

Desolation Wilderness and the South Lake Tahoe Basin

1st Edition 1980
2nd Edition 1985
3rd Edition August 1996
4th Edition September 2003
  3rd printing April 2008

Front cover photo copyright © 2005 by Mark E. Vollmer
Interior photos and drawings, except where noted, by Jeffrey P. Schaffer
Maps: Ben Pease, based on information from United States Geologic Survey
  Glacier map digitized by Jaan Hitt. Topographic maps and information sup-
  plied by the author. Wilderness Press also publishes a separate full-size map
  of the Desolation Wilderness area.
Cover design: Lisa Pletka
Book design: Jaan Hitt

ISBN 978-0-89997-328-9
UPC 7-19609-97328-7

Manufactured in the United States of America

Published by: **Wilderness Press**
               1200 5th Street
               Berkeley, CA 94710
               (800) 443-7227; FAX (510) 558-1696
               info@wildernesspress.com
               www.wildernesspress.com
Visit our website for a complete listing of our books and for ordering information.

Cover photo: Ancient juniper at Heather Lake, Desolation Wilderness
Frontispiece: Heather Lake, Pyramid Peak (far left) and the Crystal Range

SAFETY NOTICE: Although Wilderness Press and the author have made every
attempt to ensure that the information in this book is accurate at press time, they
are not responsible for any loss, damage, injury, or inconvenience that may occur
to anyone while using this book. You are responsible for your own safety and
health while in the wilderness. The fact that a trail is described in this book does
not mean that it will be safe for you. Be aware that trail conditions can change
from day to day. Always check local conditions and know your own limitations.

Read This

Hiking in the backcountry entails unavoidable risk that every hiker assumes and must be aware of and respect. The fact that a trail is described in this book is not a guarantee that it will be safe for you. Trails vary greatly in difficulty and in the degree of conditioning and agility one needs to enjoy them safely. On some hikes, routes may have changed or conditions may have deteriorated since the descriptions were written. Also, trail conditions can change even from day to day, owing to weather and other factors. A trail that is safe on a dry day or for a highly conditioned, agile, properly equipped hiker may be completely unsafe for someone else or unsafe under adverse weather conditions. You can minimize your risks on the trail by being knowledgeable, prepared, and alert. There is not space in this book for a general treatise on safety in the mountains, but there are a number of good books and public courses on the subject and you should take advantage of them to increase your knowledge. Just as important, you should always be aware of your own limitations and of conditions existing when and where you are hiking. If conditions are dangerous, or if you are not prepared to deal with them safely, choose a different hike! It's better to have wasted a drive than to be the subject of a mountain rescue. These warnings are not intended to scare you off the trails. Millions of people have safe and enjoyable hikes every year. However, one element of the beauty, freedom, and excitement of the wilderness is the presence of risks that do not confront us at home. When you hike you assume those risks. They can be met safely, but only if you exercise your own independent judgment and common sense.

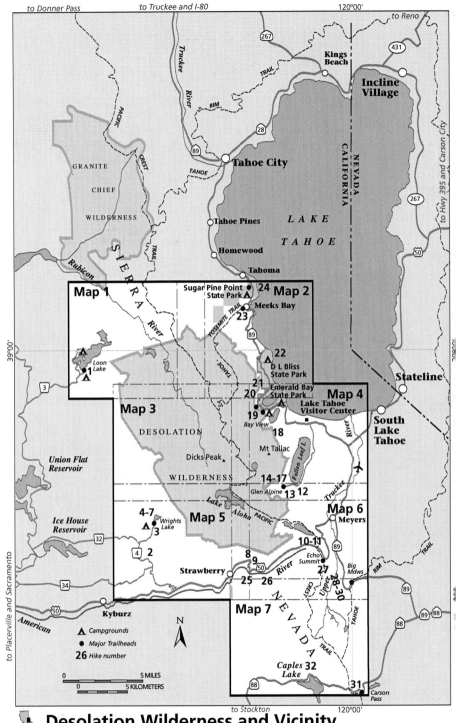

Desolation Wilderness and Vicinity

Contents

Dedication

For my wife and daughter, Bonnie and Mary Anne

Preface

Most of this book's hikes were taken from a section of The Tahoe Sierra (1975 edition) that was entitled "Trails of the Highway 50 Region." I hiked and mapped the trails in that section in 1974, accompanied and aided on many days by Kenneth Ng. In 1976, 1978, and 1979 I rehiked some of those trails plus other Tahoe trails not found in that book. With this new information I compiled Desolation Wilderness, which was read in manuscript form by Nathan Leising of the Lake Tahoe Basin Management Unit of the US Forest Service. Since then I have done trail scouting every couple of years, the last year being 1995. The natural-history chapter has evolved with time, especially the geology subchapter. Over the years I came to realize that there were problems with the standard interpretations. In my lengthy Ph.D. dissertation (third draft, 1995—later much abridged), I was able to demonstrate that virtually everything written about uplift and glaciation of the range was incorrect. The biology subchapter has changed much less.

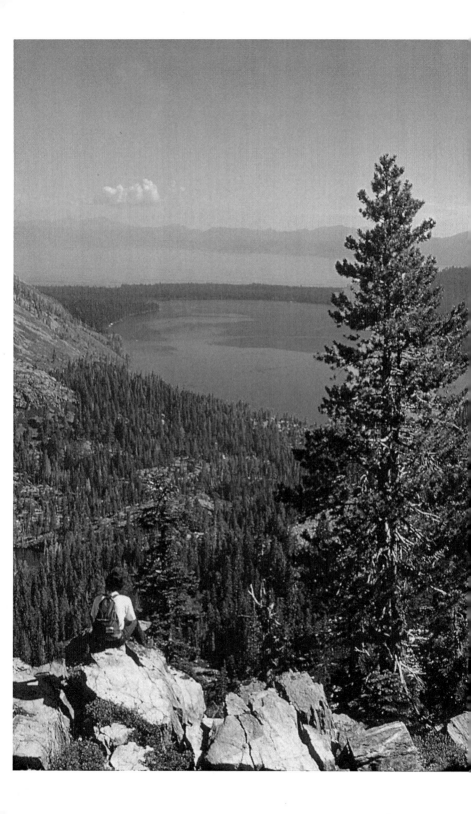

Chapter 1	# The Country

One of California's most popular hiking areas, dominated by Desolation Wilderness, stands above the southwest shore of giant, mountain-rimmed Lake Tahoe. To the north a smaller hiking area, dominated by Granite Chief Wilderness, siphons some visitors to the sub-alpine country west of Tahoe's northwest shore, but this loss hardly makes a dent in the summertime "urban population" found in Desolation Wilderness. By the late 1970s this wilderness had grown so much in popularity that the Forest Service began to limit the number of backpackers entering it. Flying over the majestic Lake Tahoe Basin, you would expect most of the lands below you to be laced with scenic, public hiking trails. This, unfortunately, is not true, for the mountains north, south, and east above Lake Tahoe are, like most of the lake's shoreline, in private hands. Hence the brunt of the hiking use congregates in Desolation Wilderness and the adjacent mountain lands above the south shore of Lake Tahoe. Most of these lands are shown on the USGS *Fallen Leaf Lake* 15-minute topographic map, and this map, in updated form, can be found on pages 180-193. Trails, however, don't stop at the map's edge; rather they continue out to their trailheads. Hence the author has added some sections to this primary map in order to show all of this book's described trails in their entirety. These trails have been consolidated into 32 hikes found in four areas: Desolation Wilderness, Emerald Bay, South Fork American River, and Upper Truckee River.

Desolation Wilderness

This book's star attraction is compact Desolation Wilderness, which is certainly northern California's most accessible wilderness. It's about a 3-hour drive from the San Francisco Bay Area, a 2-hour drive from Sacramento, and a few minutes' drive from South Lake Tahoe. This 100-square-mile roadless area stands as an island of "primitive solitude" hemmed in on all sides by civilization's demands. Logging and grazing occur close to its western and northern borders, while widespread development west and south of South Lake Tahoe cause the exclusion of Cascade, Fallen Leaf, and Echo lakes. To the south Highway 50 and its developments prevent union with southern mountain lands.

Compact it is

Averaging 12½ miles long by 8 miles wide, this wilderness can be traversed in any direction by a strong hiker in a day or less. Because it is so compact and readily accessible, it is too crowded to be considered a wilderness in the strict sense of the word. Although wilderness areas should be pristine havens for solitude, don't expect to find any unless you get off the beaten path, which requires mountain skills. And pristine it's not: dozens of lakes have low dams, through the 1900s several hundred cattle invaded the west side in late summer, and today some visitors still leave traces of their presence (latrines would be most welcome at popular sites). Although backpackers are limited to 700 per day, day hikers are unlimited. Both groups need wilderness permits, and those caught without them may be cited (see Chapter 2's section on **Wilderness Permits**). With all these visitors treading the trails and splashing or fishing in the lakes, Desolation Wilderness is neither desolate nor wild; rather, it's best viewed as a mountain playland, an extension of the Lake Tahoe recreation scene.

And what attracts hikers to this readily accessible, triple-crested wilderness? Its Crystal Range, which is the prominent, granite crest you see when driving east up Highway 50, averages only 9500 feet in elevation, and the two crests east of it are even lower—hardly a match for central California's High Sierra. But where else can you find 130 lakes, about 90 of them named, packed into 100 square miles of mountain scenery? Although Desolation Wilderness occupies only ⅓ of the area covered by this guidebook's maps, it accounts for ⅚ of its lakes.

Like Yosemite National Park, Desolation Wilderness averages about 8000 feet in elevation, and this general elevation figure seems to be ideal for lake formation. Indeed, the great bulk of the Desolation Wilderness lakes lie between 7500 and 8300 feet, and with mountain crests averaging 9000 feet, there is sufficient relief to wrap the lakes in dramatic backdrops. Most of the landscape, like that of the High Sierra, is composed of granitic rock, differing significantly from the Sierra crests north and south of the wilderness, which are mostly composed of thick volcanic deposits. This granitic rock fractures into an array of patterns, resulting in myriad shapes of lakes, which occupy bedrock basins excavated by glaciers. Furthermore, about 15% of the landscape is metamorphic, and this belt of rock, cutting east-west across the middle of the wilderness, paints the landscape in multihued earth tones, which are magnified when reflected in the still waters of, say, Gilmore and Lois lakes.

In short, Desolation Wilderness is a mountain landscape that incorporates in a very small area most of the best features found in the High Sierra. It is prime lake country, ranging from 6140 to 9983 feet in elevation. It is high enough to avoid the oppressive summer heat found to the west, yet low enough for the hiker to get by with light clothing (though extra clothes and emergency gear should always be taken). Its mountains rise high enough to make them a strong attraction, yet low enough to provide relatively easy accessibility through the countryside.

The trails of Desolation Wilderness are described in Hikes 1-20 and 23. The hikes are arranged in a counterclockwise arc, starting at Loon Lake, near the wilderness' northwest corner, and circling around to General Creek Campground (the start of Hike 24), near its northeast corner. Hikes 21, 22, and 24, along this arc, lie just east of the wilderness. Hikes 3 and 12 are also outside the wilderness, though each can be linked with a trail leading into it.

Several trails are omitted. Beyond the topographic map's west edge and below McConnell Peak are trails to Shadow Lake, outside the wilderness, and Forni Lake, within it. From the latter a primitive trail climbs east to the saddle west of Highland Lake. This is a quick, though potentially dangerous, way to that lake, and is for accomplished mountaineers only. The primitive trail climbs north to nearby Tells Peak, a worthy goal, but then makes a lengthy, near-crest, sometimes cryptic descent to the Rubicon Trail. Finally, from a trail's end above Cascade Lake, on the east side of the wilderness, a fairly popular, though potentially dangerous, mountaineers' route climbs to Snow and Azure lakes.

The best period to visit is about August 5-20, when lakes are usually at their maximum temperatures and the days are warm. Before late June only Hike 1 is sufficiently snow-free for enjoyable hiking. By early to mid-July, however, most of the trails are hikeable and passes open, while the lakes, depending on their elevation and surrounding topography, are beginning to warm. Except for the

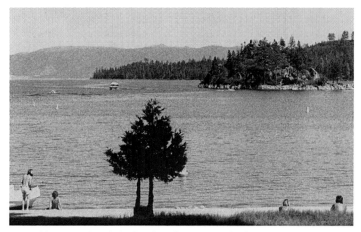

Emerald Bay's Vikingsholm beach and Fannette Island

low Hike 1 terrain, mosquitoes are an extreme nuisance almost everywhere through late July, so bring a tent and an effective repellent. August, being the most pleasant month, is the most crowded one, and wilderness quotas for overnighters can fill rapidly. After mid-September, use decreases quickly and, except for an occasional, usually mild storm, the days are quite pleasant even though the nights can be freezing. During week days, in particular, you may be alone in watching autumn paint the deciduous vegetation in warm hues. However, hunters can abound in late September and early October, that is, during deer season. About mid-October the days become too cool for most hikers, and about then or soon after, a major storm dumps sufficient snow to keep trails buried until the next June.

Emerald Bay

A national scenic treasure such as Lake Tahoe should be totally accessible to the public. Unfortunately, most of its shore is privately owned, thereby causing the public to crowd the lake's relatively few public beaches. Lester Beach, in D. L. Bliss State Park, is one such beach. However, most of this park's shoreline is seldom visited, and for the bather seeking relative solitude, Hike 22, from the Lester Beach area south to Emerald Bay, offers shoreline access at a number of points. Hike 21 drops to Emerald Bay State Park's Vikingsholm beach, Tahoe's only substantial public beach to which one must hike. On summer weekends its popularity is limited only by available parking space. Because you can reach

Vikingsholm Beach in a 15-minute walk, it is a good place to refresh yourself after a strenuous Desolation Wilderness hike. Of course, Lake Tahoe's public beaches require even less effort. Both Emerald Bay and Lake Tahoe are chilly by most people's standards. At best they warm to the mid-60s by August through mid-September; to the low 60s or lower before then.

South Fork American River

The terrain just south of Highway 50 resembles Desolation Wilderness in that it is mostly granite and has been somewhat glaciated. But one glance at map 7 tells you this area is quite different—it is almost lakeless. Although past glaciers filled every canyon from the Upper Truckee River canyon west to the Strawberry Creek canyon, sizable lakes developed in only two unlikely locations. Lake Audrian, near Echo Summit, lies in a shallow trough that was slightly eroded by an overflowing lobe of the giant Upper Truckee River glacier. Near the middle of the south base of the map is Cody Lake, which lies on a granitic bench halfway up a Cody Creek side canyon. Both lakes lack good trails to them.

Only four trails, combined into three hikes, are described in this section of the book. Hike 25 guides you to Lovers Leap in under an hour's time. From this summit you can *carefully* look down its steep northwest face, which provides some of the best and most challenging climbing routes found in the entire Lake Tahoe area. Nonclimbers will appreciate the splendid views up- and down-canyon, which include a head-on view of the prominent lateral moraines lining the sides of Pyramid Creek canyon. This Lovers Leap Trail is usually hikeable from early June through mid-October. Hike 26, the Sayles Canyon and Bryan Meadow trails, offers neither lakes nor views, just pleasant forest punctuated by two mountain meadows. Lacking Desolation Wilderness attractions, this hike also lacks its crowds. Only nature lovers need apply. Technically, Hike 27, a stretch of the Pacific Crest Trail, lies in the Upper Truckee River drainage, but is included here because it crosses similar terrain. Both 26 and 27 usually are open from early July through mid-October, mid-to-late July being best for flowers, August best for ideal temperatures and minimal mosquitoes.

Upper Truckee River

Today's Upper Truckee River did not cut the mammoth canyon it now occupies. Late in the days of the dinosaurs, a fault formed and the canyon originated along it, deepening and widening over millions of years. More recently, glaciers flowed through it, but they did little more than create shallow basins now filled with lakes. Hikes 29-32 provide routes to the four largest lakes, Hikes 31-32 being particularly scenic. All the basin's lakes are at least partly rimmed with granitic bedrock and in that respect they resemble the lakes of Desolation Wilderness. However, in each of these lake hikes you tread on some volcanic soil, and, with volcanic rocks lining the basin's walls, your impressions of this scenery will differ from those of any Desolation Wilderness hike. Hike 28, along an abandoned, lakeless, historic road, perhaps will appeal only to history buffs and those in search of exercise. Still, it can be used to complete a loop trip to all four lakes. Take Hike 29 to Dardanelles Lake, visit Round, Meiss, and Showers lakes (Hikes 30-31), then trek north on the Pacific Crest Trail (Hike 27 in reverse), taking the alternate route to near the top end of Hike 28. This you descend in reverse toward the original trailhead, which, if you're willing to ford the Upper Truckee River, is only 100 yards from Hike 28's trailhead. Otherwise, add ½ mile along roads. Subalpine Showers Lake, due to its high elevation, may be partly snow-lined until early August, and never warms for comfortable swimming. The other lakes are worth visiting from July through September.

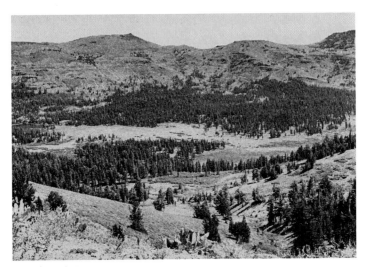

Upper Truckee canyon

Chapter 2

Hiking in the Tahoe Area

B efore delving into this guidebook's 32 hikes, you might first read this chapter, which covers information you should know for a safe, enjoyable, and informative excursion. If you're too anxious to head up to Desolation Wilderness and can't take the time to read this chapter, at least read the sections on **Wilderness Permits** and on **Minimum Impact**. Doing so will save you a lot of time and frustration, and you'll avoid possibly getting cited for entering the wilderness without a permit.

This Guidebook's 32 Hikes

Hike Organization

The trails shown in this book's 7 topographic maps are consolidated into and described in 32 hikes. These hikes fall into two broad divisions (see trailhead map). If you were to drive counterclockwise around the perimeter of Desolation Wilderness, north of Highway 50, you would encounter Hikes 1-24 in the order they appear in this book. If you were to drive clockwise around the mountain lands south of Highway 50, you would encounter Hikes 25-32 in their proper order.

On the counterclockwise loop, Hikes 1-7 cover trails along the western section of Desolation Wilderness, while Hikes 8-11 start near the wilderness' south edge. Hikes 8 and 9 describe features near Lake Aloha while Hikes 10 and 11 describe features seen as you hike north through the middle of the wilderness. Hikes 12-20 cover trails around the southeast part of the wilderness, while 23-24 cover those in or near its northeast part. Hikes 21 and 22 cover trails of Emerald Bay, which lies just east of the wilderness.

On the clockwise loop, Hikes 25-27 cover trails south of Highway 50, from Lovers Leap east to Echo Summit. Hikes 28-30 start from Upper Truckee Road (and Highway 89), while Hikes 31-32 start on or near Highway 88. Hikes 27-32 lead into the Upper Truckee River basin.

Hike Description

For each hike, directions are given to its trailhead and mileages are given to its main destinations. These destinations, usually lakes, are listed because many visitors will walk only partway along a hike, and they will want to know the mileage of *their* planned excursion. For example, not many people will follow 13.8-mile Hike 1 to its end just past Camper Flat; rather, most will proceed no farther than Rubicon Reservoir, 8.3 miles from the trailhead.

The hike description naturally gives all appropriate trail directions, but it does more than that. It also mentions, and sometimes elaborates on, the natural features seen along the trail. Photographs show many of these features, and may help you decide which hike to take. While this book emphasizes geographical features, which largely draw the outdoor crowds to this area, it minimizes the biological features—fish and wildflowers in particular. Suffice it to say that almost every lake you'll encounter is stocked with trout. Experience shows that whenever a guidebook states that a lake has excellent fishing, anglers will rush to it, rapidly downgrading its fishing status to poor. Also, in the past, fishing guides have played havoc with the Department of Fish and Game's stocking program. Wildflowers, mentioned in Chapter 3, are beautiful and are the prime attractions for a few hikers, but they are rarely mentioned in trail descriptions because they are so ephemeral. Some bloom early, others late, and the kind *and* amount of flowers you'll see depend on what month you hike in. And their numbers can vary considerably from year to year. For maximum wildflower exposure, hike in July—which unfortunately is usually a time mosquitoes are quite abundant. Both peak in early summer, taking advantage of the abundant snowmelt water.

Selecting a Hike

Chapter 1 introduces you to this area and its hikes, but more should be said. Except for Hikes 9, 25, 26, and 28, all visit one or more lakes. Hence, if lakes are what you have in mind, you have quite a selection from which to choose. The following table lists this area's major lakes in order of increasing distance from a trailhead. It lists the shortest distance to each lake, which isn't always the easiest route. Hike 8's 2.4-mile climb to Ropi Lake is certainly more strenuous and dangerous than Hike 10's 4.5-mile climb to it (7.0 miles without water taxi). Likewise, hikes of a given length can vary greatly in difficulty. While almost anyone can hike the 4.5 miles to Spider Lake with little effort, some people trying to hike the 4.5 miles to Upper Velma Lake may turn back in agonizing despair. In sum, the lake-distance table just gives you an overall, simplified view of this area's lakes; consult this book's topo maps and the appropriate hike (its introduction and description) for a better impression of the route that interests you. If you're in average shape you can day-hike to all lakes under 5 miles except Dicks, Fontanillis, and Velma lakes (all in Hike 20, which makes a very steep climb). However, many hikers, anglers in particular, prefer to backpack to any lake more than one mile from its trailhead.

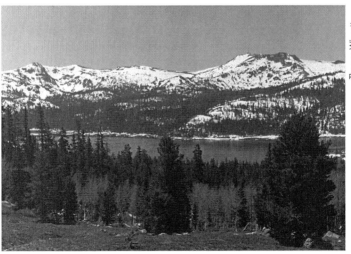

Caples Lake

Table of Shortest Distances to This Area's Lakes

Longer routes to these lakes are omitted. The number in each set of parentheses refers to the hike that goes to that lake in the shortest distance. Hike 10 mileages assume you've taken the water taxi, which saves 2.5 miles. Hike 8 provides the shortest way in to Avalanche, Pitt, and Ropi lakes, but it is too dangerous for many hikers, who should take Hike 10 instead.

Miles	Lakes
0.5	Lower Angora Lake (12)
0.6	Beauty Lake (4)
0.8	Upper Angora Lake (12), Lake Tahoe, at Emerald Bay's Vikingsholm beach (21)
1.0	Eagle Lake (20)
1.1	Granite Lake (19)
1.3	Tamarack Lake (10)
1.6	Ralston Lake (10), Cagwin Lake (10)
1.7	Triangle Lake (10), Floating Island Lake (18)
1.8	Bloodsucker Lake (3)
1.9	Avalanche Lake (8)
2.0	Pitt Lake (8)
2.1	Grouse Lake (5), Showers Lake (32)
2.5	Ropi Lake (8), Cathedral Lake (18)
2.6	Hemlock Lake (5), Lake Margery (10), Grass Lake (14)
2.7	Lower Twin Lake (5), Lake Lucille (10)
2.8	Lake of the Woods (10)
2.9	Meiss Lake (32)
3.0	Smith Lake (5)
3.1	Upper Twin Lake (5), Boomerang Lake (5), Round Lake (30)
3.3	Island Lake (5), Lake Aloha (10)
3.6	Richardson Lake (11)
3.8	Gertrude Lake (6)
3.9	Tyler Lake(6)
4.0	Dardanelles Lake (30)

Miles	Lakes
4.1	Loon Lake, at its Pleasant Campground (1), Susie Lake (15)
4.2	Lake LeConte (10), Gilmore Lake (17)
4.3	Dicks Lake (20)
4.4	Middle Velma Lake (20)
4.5	Spider Lake (1), Upper Velma Lake (20)
4.6	Maud Lake (7), Lake Genevieve (23)
4.7	Pearl Lake (4)
4.8	Half Moon Lake (16)
4.9	Lake Sylvia (2), Fontanillis Lake (20), Crag Lake (23)
5.0	Lyons Lake (2)
5.2	Heather Lake (15)
5.3	Lake Winifred(l)
5.5	Alta Morris Lake (16)
5.7	Hidden Lake (23)
5.9	Barrett Lake (4), Shadow Lake (23)
6.1	Buck Island Lake (1)
6.2	Lake Doris (7)
6.3	Lawrence Lake (4), Stony Ridge Lake (23)
6.7	Rockbound Lake (1), Lake No. 5 (4)
6.8	Lake No. 9 (4), Clyde Lake (10)
6.9	Top Lake (4)
7.3	Lake No. 4 (4), Lake Lois (7), Duck Lake (24)
7.5	Lost Lake (24)
7.6	Lake No. 3 (4)
8.1	Rubicon Lake (23)
8.2	Fox Lake (1)
8.3	Rubicon Reservoir (1)
8.6	Lake Schmidell (7)
9.8	Lower Leland Lake (7)
10.6	McConnell Lake (7)
11.8	Horseshoe Lake (7)
12.0	4-Q Lakes(7)
12.3	Lake Zitella (7)
13.5	Highland Lake (7)

A few hikes climb to prominent summits

These are Hike 9 (Ralston Peak, 4.6 miles), Hike 13 (Echo Peak, 3.6 miles), Hike 17 (Mt. Tallac, 6.0 miles), Hike 18 (Mt. Tallac, 4.6 miles), and Hike 25 (Lovers Leap, 1.4 miles). If you take the Echo Lakes water taxi, then Hike 10 provides the shortest route to Ralston and Echo peaks, 4.3 and 2.6 miles respectively. All summits provide rewarding views, the one from Mt. Tallac being, in the author's opinion, the best. Of course, you needn't climb to a mountaintop to get a superlative view; these exist along many trails covered by this guide. Mountaineers may want to go cross-country to climb trailless peaks, Pyramid Peak in particular (see Hike 2). And most rock climbers know that Tahoe's best climbing cliff is Lovers Leap (see Hike 25). Where other climbing opportunities exist, this guide identifies them.

Perhaps you have friends who've hiked in this area, and they can tell you their favorite trails and lakes. Some of the choicest spots are off the trail, and these I leave for your own discovery. Discovery is, after all, an important part of the wilderness experience. After you peruse this book's hikes, odds are you'll select a hike into Desolation Wilderness. To enter it, you'll need a wilderness permit.

Wilderness Permits

During the 1960s, backpacking, with its new, lightweight technology, came of age, and hikers proliferated throughout the Sierra Nevada. By the time Desolation Wilderness was officially created in late 1969, it was already crowded. In 1971 the Forest Service began a permit system, in part to study visitor use and impact. The Forest Service determined that the wilderness' optimum capacity was about 2100 persons at one time, which was considerably less than what could be found on a typical summer day. In 1978 the Forest Service began a quota system in which it limited the number of overnight users. *Wilderness permits are required for both overnight users and day users. If you enter the wilderness without a permit, you could be issued a violation notice by a patrolling ranger.*

For the latest information, use the internet. The Forest Service's Region 5 internet address is **www.r5.fs.fed.us.** Once there, you can click on the appropriate national forest (Eldorado). For the Lake Tahoe Basin Management Unit, reach it directly at **www.r5.fs.fed.us/ltbmu;** for the Eldorado National Forest Information Center, **www.r5.fs.fed.us./eldorado**. Overnight Desolation Wilderness visitors only: you have to pay for wilderness permits, $5 per person per day for the first two days (additional days are free).

When

Wilderness permits are necessary *every day* of the year, even in the dead of winter when no one may be present but you. For a true wilderness experience, *experienced* hikers should visit the area when it is snowbound, from about November through May. Then, the traces of man lie beneath the snow and solitude reigns supreme.

How many

The Forest Service dispenses permits for up to 700 over-night users per day. Up to 350 persons per day can reserve them, and knowledgeable users do just that. The quota system is in effect from the Friday before Memorial Day through September 30. For the rest of the year the use is sufficiently less that a quota system is unnecessary. At present the number of day users is unrestricted, but because this policy may change, call one of the offices listed below to check on current requirements.

Where

You can reserve a wilderness permit by writing, phoning or visiting the Forest Service *within* 90 days of the start of your proposed hike. (The Forest Service prefers you get a permit in person.) Reserved permits are mailed to you, although any changes to reserved permits must be made in person at one of the offices. There are three offices for this. If you plan to enter the wilderness anywhere west of the Sierra crest (i.e., west of Echo Summit), stop at the **Pacific Ranger District** located 4 miles east of Pollock Pines on Highway 50. Their address is 7887 Highway 50, Pollock Pines, CA 95726. The phone number is (530) 647-5415. For east-side entry, stop at the **Lake Tahoe Visitor Center.** It is located on the right side of Highway 89 about 3 miles north-west of the Highway 50/89 split in South Lake Tahoe. The center's entrance road is just 150 yards past the Fallen Leaf Road. The phone number is (530) 543-2674. Alternatively, you could stop at the **Lake Tahoe Basin Management Unit**, which is locat-ed in the Plaza 89 center at 870 Emerald Bay Road (a.k.a. Highway 89) in South Lake Tahoe, 0.3 mile northwest of the split. Their address is 35 College Drive, South Lake Tahoe, CA 96150. The phone number is (530) 543-2600.

If you complete a wilderness permit application by mail or fax, you will have to supply your name, address, phone number, trailhead entry and exit points, trip dates, number in hiking party, and proposed hiking itinerary (for example: 8/11, Wrights Lake trailhead to Lake Schmidell; 8/12, Lake Schmidell to Middle Velma Lake; 8/13, Middle Velma Lake to Lake Aloha; 8/14, Lake Aloha to Lake Doris; 8/15, Lake Doris to Wrights Lake trailhead).

Day users have the option of obtaining a wilderness permit at one of the three offices mentioned above or at their trailhead. Permits are available at the major trailheads, but not at the minor ones. Furthermore, on busy days popular trailheads can run out of permits. Consequently, you may have to drive to a nearby trailhead for a permit or head out to one of the three offices. If permits are not available at your trailhead and you enter the wilderness without one, you can be cited by a patrolling ranger.

Campgrounds

Because hikers often stay at campgrounds either before or after their hikes, this guidebook lists campgrounds, grouping them by hike and listing them in the order you would encounter them. For example, those driving to the Hike 1 trailhead would encounter Sunset Campground first and Loon Lake Campground last.

Unless termed "private," all campgrounds are administered by government agencies. During the summer, many of the campgrounds fill up, especially on weekends, so you should make reservations well in advance (ideally, 2 to 4 months). **Only some of the *public* campgrounds are on a reservation system, and these are identified with an asterisk (*).** For Forest Service campground reservations, contact the National Recreation Reservation Service at (800) 280-2267 or www.reserveusa.com; for State Park campground reservations (Emerald Bay, D. L. Bliss, General Creek), use (800) 444-7275 or www.parks.ca.gov.

In the early 2000s public campgrounds generally cost about 15 to 20 dollars per day. Rates for private campgrounds cost about double, but provide hot showers and other amenities. All private campgrounds tend to be noisy because they are next to a busy highway or, for Tahoe Valley Campground, because sporadic noise comes from aircraft climbing overhead from nearby Lake Tahoe Airport. On the other hand, because public campgrounds lack electrical hookups, recreational vehicles in them often have annoying generators operating. Additionally, from the author's experience, rowdy campers frequent the cheaper (i.e., public)

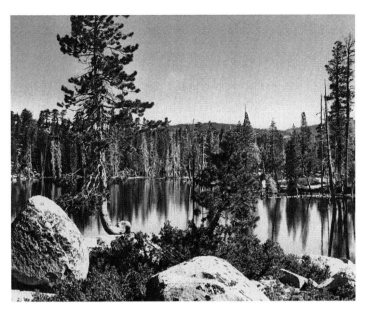

Spider Lake

campgrounds. (Most private campgrounds are well patrolled and do not tolerate disturbance; public ones tend to be under-patrolled or not patrolled at all).

Hike 1

*Sunset Campground, Wench Creek Campground, *Yellowjacket Campground:** All three are larger campgrounds around Union Valley Reservoir, just west of Forest Route 3. **South Fork Campground:** Just 0.1 mile past the Forest Route 1 junction, branch left, go 0.8 mile, and branch right 0.1 mile. ***Loon Lake Campground:** Near the Hike 1 trailhead.

Hikes 2-7

*Wrights Lake Campground:** By the trailheads for Hikes 3-7.

Hikes 8-11

Lake Tahoe KOA (private; (530) 577-3693): On Highway 50 immediately southwest of the Upper Truckee Road junction.

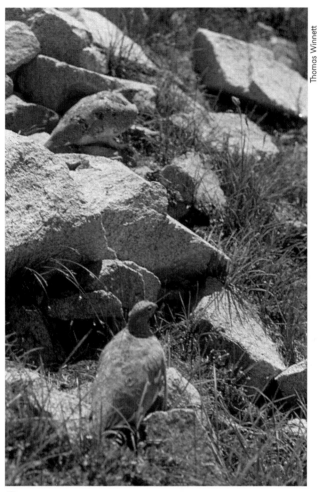

Thomas Winnett

Grouse

Hikes 12-18

Tahoe Valley Campground (private; (530) 541-2222): One block east of Highway 50, just 0.4 mile south of the Highways 50/89 split in South Lake Tahoe. **Richardson's Resort** (private; (530) 541-1801; (800) 544-1801): On Highway 89 about 2½ miles northwest of the Highways 50/89 split in South Lake Tahoe and ½ mile before Fallen Leaf Road. ***Fallen Leaf Campground:** 0.5 mile south on Fallen Leaf Road.

Hikes 19-22

*Emerald Bay State Park (two camping areas): Northeast slopes above head of Emerald Bay. Bay View Campground (24-hour limit): Above Emerald Bay. *D. L. Bliss State Park (five camping areas): Along park road down to the Hike 22 trailhead.

Hikes 23-24

*Meeks Bay Campground: Just 230 yards south of the Hike 23 trailhead. Meeks Bay Resort (private; (530) 525-7242): Just 250 yards north of the Hike 23 trailhead. *General Creek Campground (Sugar Pine Point State Park): By the Hike 24 trailhead. *William Kent Campground: By William Kent Visitor Center, 2.2 miles south of Tahoe City.

Hikes 25-30

Same campgrounds listed under Hikes 8-11 plus undeveloped campsites (no fee) along road descending from the Big Meadow trailhead (Hike 30).

Hikes 31-32

Caples Lake Campground: On Highway 88 opposite Caples Lake Resort. Schneider Camping Area (primitive campground without water; no fee): 0.4 mile before the Hike 32 trailhead.

Backpacking and Day Hiking

General

Most of the hikes in this book can be done as day hikes rather than as overnight hikes, although you may want to take more than one day to do many of them. Generally, however, each requires very little planning and preparation. Novices to backpacking can learn the art by reading a copy of *Backpacking Basics* (Wilderness Press).

Because detailed, updated maps are included in this guide, mileage figures within the text are kept at a minimum. There are, however, numerous instances where vertical distance in feet and horizontal distance in yards are given. The first is given to tell you how much you will have to climb, thereby informing those who like easy hikes what they're in for. The second distance has a more practical reason: some trail junctions can be missed if poorly signed or if snow still covers the trail. Therefore, potentially hard-to-find junctions are identified by their distance from the nearest identifiable feature—often a creek crossing. Yards are given because they approximately equal long strides—when in doubt, the hiker can pace off the distance.

Your progress along a trail is often measured with respect to a prominent feature in the landscape, such as a mountain or a hill above you. On this guide's topographic maps, many unnamed high points are identified by an **X**, which marks the point, and a number, which gives the elevation. This guide refers to these high points as peaks—for example, peak 9224.

Some trails in this guide are potentially hard to follow in a few spots. Others may have lingering snow patches that hide them. For both, your route can usually be found by watching for blazes or ducks that mark the trail. A *blaze* is a conspicuous man-made scar on a tree trunk that results from the removal of a patch or two of bark. A *duck* is one or more small rocks placed on a larger rock in such a way that the placement is obviously unnatural.

Minimal-Impact Hiking

If thousands of hikers walk through a mountain landscape, with its fragile soils, they are almost bound to degrade it. The following suggestions are offered in the hope they will reduce human imprint on the landscape, thus keeping it attractive for those who might follow.

First, if you're healthy enough to make an outdoor trip into a wilderness area, you're in good enough condition to do so on foot. Leave horses behind. (However, most hunters who enter Desolation Wilderness and other mountain areas in late September and early October will certainly object to carrying a deer out on their shoulders.) One horse may do more damage than a dozen backpackers. It will contribute at least as much excrement as all of them, but moreover, it will do so indiscriminately, sometimes in creeks or at lakeshores. Another problem with horses is that they can transform meadow trails into muddy ruts, particularly in early season. And they selectively graze the meadows, impacting certain native plants. For example, only 30 years after Yosemite Valley was set aside as a state park in 1864, its luxuriant native grasses and wildflowers were reduced to about one-fourth their original number, largely replaced by hardier, less showy alien species. Also impacting meadows, though probably to a lesser degree, are grazing animals, especially cattle. In comparison, the relatively few horses have made only a minor impact. Occasionally it's the riders rather than the horses that are a problem. It's so easy to pack in food for a feast and leave garbage, cans, and bottles littering the campsite. If you do bring stock animals into Desolation Wilderness, it is recommended that you take supplemental feed, and you're not allowed to tie or picket them in any meadow or within 200 feet of water.

If at all possible, day-hike rather than overnight-hike. As was mentioned earlier, you can make easy-to-moderate day hikes to over half of the Desolation Wilderness lakes, and the same applies to the lakes outside the wilderness. Actually, if you're *really* in shape, there's no reason you can't day-hike to *any* lake under 10 miles away and *enjoy* it (and mountaineers, using cross-country shortcuts, can reach them all). Such a hike should take about 6 hours or less to walk, plus the time spent relaxing at spots. Anglers will object, since fishing is best around dawn and dusk. Who wants to get up at three in the morning to fish a lake at dawn? For them, backpacking is a must. Still, trout-stocked mountain lakes are an unnatural phenomenon, and some naturalists question continuance of the stocking program.

Why do day-hikers have less impact on the environment? For one thing, they usually use toilets near trailheads rather than soil near lakes. Seven hundred backpackers in Desolation Wilderness contribute about a ton of excrement *per week*, and the bulk of this is within 100 yards of a lake, stream, or trail. Whereas horse and cattle excrement, lying on the ground, decomposes rapidly, buried human excrement takes longer. Excrement can lead to deterioration of a lake's water quality. Always defecate at least 100 feet away from any lake or stream, and the Forest Service recommends you bury feces 6-8 inches deep. *However, environmentally conscious campers will carry out both toilet paper and feces, and then dispose of them properly after reaching the trailhead.*

If, in order to have a satisfactory wilderness experience, you decide to backpack, please consider the following advice, which is specifically aimed at those visiting Desolation Wilderness, but is applicable to all overnighters in the mountains.

1. Pack out all trash, including toilet paper. Popular lakes can receive over a thousand visitors during a summer, and there is a limit to how much paper can be buried.

2. Don't build a campfire unless you absolutely have to do so, as in an emergency. They are *prohibited* in Desolation Wilderness. Downed wood is already too scarce, and cutting or defacing standing vegetation, whether living or dead, is prohibited. Use a stove instead, which cooks meals faster, leaves pots and pans

cleaner, and saves downed wood for the soil's organisms, which are consumed by animals. Campfires can leave an unsightly mess and, as the snowpack melts, campfire ashes can be carried into lakes, reducing their water quality. If you are backpacking *outside* the wilderness, you'll need a *campfire permit* if you intend to build a fire. Get one at a Forest Service office. A campfire permit requires you to carry a shovel. If you don't build any fires but use only a gas stove, then you can leave the shovel behind, but will still need the permit.

3. Don't pollute lakes and streams by washing clothes or dishes in them or throwing fish entrails into them. And don't lather up in them, even with biodegradable soap. *All* soaps pollute. Do your washing and pot scrubbing well away from lakes and streams, and bury fish entrails ashore rather than throw them back into the water.

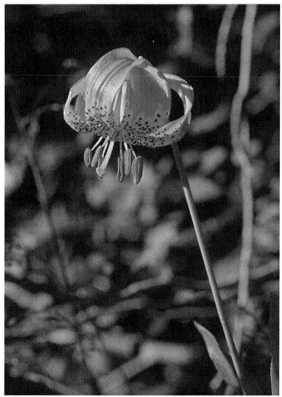

Leopard lily

4. Set up camp at least 100 feet from streams, trails, and lakeshores. At some lakes this may be practically impossible, and then you must be extremely careful not to degrade the environment. Always camp on mineral soil (or perhaps even on bedrock, if you've brought sufficient padding), but never in meadows or other soft, vegetated areas. It's best to use an existing site rather than to brush out a new one, which would result in one more human mark upon the landscape.

5. Leave your campsite clean. Don't leave scraps of food behind, for it only attracts mice, bears, and other camp marauders. If you can carry it in, you can carry it out. After all, your pack is lighter on the way out and the trail is probably downhill.

6. Don't build structures. Rock walls, large fireplaces, and bough beds were fine in John Muir's time, but not today. There are just too many humans on this planet, and one goes into the wilderness for a bit of solitude away from them. The hiker shouldn't have to be confronted with continual reminders of human presence. Leave the wilderness at least as pure as you found it.

7. Noise and loud conversations, like motor vehicles and mountain bikes, are prohibited. Have some consideration for other campers in the vicinity. Also, camp far enough away from others to assure privacy to both them and you.

8. Dogs are allowed in the wilderness, but the Forest Service strongly recommends you leave them home. If you bring one, it must be kept under control.

Regardless of whether you are day-hiking or backpacking, you should observe the following advice.

1. The smaller your party, the better. In Desolation Wilderness overnight groups are limited to 12 persons, and in it you should avoid the most popular trails if your group is 8 or more. These trails are in Hikes 5-7, 10-11, 14-17, and 20. If you do have a large party, you might consider camping outside the wilderness. Lakes outside the wilderness that can handle large groups are: Spider and Buck Island lakes (Hike 1), Barrett Lake (Hike 4), Richardson Lake (Hike 11), Lost Lake (Hike 24), Round Lake (Hike 30), and Meiss Lake (Hike 30 or 32). Also try to avoid the main hiking season, which lasts from mid July through the Labor Day weekend, when lakes are warmest.

2. If you are 16 or older, you need a California fishing license to fish. The wilderness' limit is 5 trout per day, 10 in possession. You can also have up to 10 eastern brook trout—if they are 8

inches or shorter. You also need a license to hunt. Observe all regulations.

3. Destruction, injury, or disturbance to any natural feature or public property is prohibited. This includes molesting any animal, picking flowers or other plants, damaging growing trees or standing snags.

4. Smoking is not allowed while traveling through vegetated areas. You may stop and smoke in a safe place.

5. Pack and saddle animals have the right of way on trails. Hikers should get completely off the trail, on the downhill side if possible.

6. When traveling on a trail, stay on its tread. Don't cut switchbacks, since this destroys trails. When going cross-country, don't mark your route in any way. Let others find their own way.

7. Be prepared for sudden adverse weather. It's good to carry a poncho even on a sunny day hike. It can also double as a ground cloth or emergency tent. A space blanket (2 oz. light) is also useful. Some day hikes unintentionally turn into overnight trips due to injury, getting lost, or bad weather. Never climb to a summit if ominous clouds are building above it, particularly if you hear thunder in the cloudy distance. And if you see lightning, turn back.

8. The farther you are from your trailhead, the greater is the problem if you are injured, so as a rule, don't hike alone.

Giardiasis

Mountain waters sometimes contain microscopic, disease-producing organisms. One is *Giardia lamblia*, whose cystic form can be found in clear mountain streams and lakes, even if they look, smell, and taste fine. Although the disease it causes, giardiasis, can be incapacitating, it is not usually life-threatening. Symptoms usually include diarrhea, gas, nausea, loss of appetite, abdominal cramps, and bloating. These discomforts may last up to six weeks. Symptoms do not begin immediately after ingesting giardia; they may develop after you have returned home. If properly diagnosed, the disease is curable with medication prescribed by a physician. The best method of treating water is to use a portable water filter, available in many sporting-goods stores. The safest bet, however, is to day-hike and to carry your own supply of water.

Chapter 3

Natural History of the Tahoe Area

Geology

Introduction

Measuring about 22 miles long from north to south and 12 miles wide, 191-square-mile Lake Tahoe is the country's largest mountain lake. Having a depth of 1645 feet, it is surpassed only by 21-square-mile Crater Lake, with a depth of 1932 feet. Crater Lake, discovered in 1853, went on to become a national park. Lake Tahoe, discovered in 1844, was almost destroyed by the rising tide of humanity. (Lake Tahoe, once as clear as Crater Lake, now has a maximum viewing depth of about 70 feet, versus over 100 for Crater Lake.) Alas, the geologic processes responsible for creating the Lake Tahoe Basin also kept it from achieving national park status, as we'll see. The principal piece of Tahoe land preserved for public use is Desolation Wilderness, which, like Yosemite National

Park, happened to have the right geologic constituents: it was mostly granitic, it was deeply glaciated, and it lacked economically important minerals.

The geologic history presented below is very different from that of the first two editions, for I and others have done Sierran field work that negates much of what was believed as late as the 1980s. The "new geology" incorporates new interpretations on the origin and uplift of mountain ranges and on the role of glaciers in transforming their landscapes.

First Rocks

Tahoe's geological history is a youthful one by the earth's standards. When masses of magma rising through the earth's crust solidified to form the Sierra's first granites about 240 million years ago, the earth had already reached 95% of its present age. These granitic masses, known as plutons, formed not in Desolation Wilderness but rather in the southern Sierra Nevada near Walker Pass.

About 240 million years ago, the area comprising Desolation Wilderness lay just offshore from North America, the coastline located perhaps in the vicinity of Lake Tahoe. To the east, in western Nevada, was a line of volcanoes. These did not form a towering volcanic range such as the Andes, but rather developed close to sea level. Indeed, some of their flows reached the sea. Desolation Wilderness remained a very shallow part of that sea, lying under perhaps less than 50 feet of water until volcanism waned about 220 million years ago. By then the coastline had retreated at least 50 miles east of the vicinity of Lake Tahoe. About the same time, the limestone comprising the shallow sea floor of Desolation Wilderness was part of a crustal mass that began to sink between faults, transforming it rather quickly, geologically speaking, into a deep-sea floor.

For about 40 million years that environment collected sediments. These make up the Sailor Canyon formation, and are preserved as the lower third of Desolation Wilderness' Mt. Tallac roof pendant (a remnant of older rocks atop granitic bedrock). Today this 5000-foot-thick band of sediments occurs mostly along the floor and lower slopes of Rubicon Valley from near the junction of the Schmidell and Rubicon River trails up-canyon to about ½ mile south of Camper Flat.

Between about 180 and 163 million years ago our area underwent change. The sea floor was raised, and some of the upper sediments of the Sailor Canyon formation were eroded and redeposited elsewhere. Atop this formation there developed the thick

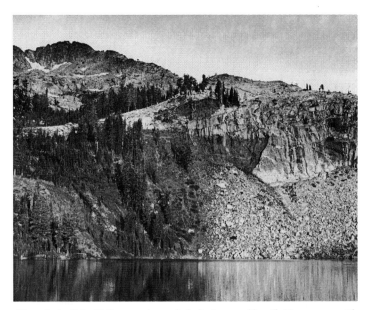

Above Lake Schmidell's west shore, dark diorite or gabbro (left) contrasts with light grandiorite. The latter breaks apart to form blocky talus, which supports far fewer plants.

Tuttle Lake formation, which accounts for the upper two thirds of the roof pendant. The lower part of the formation is composed mostly of chaotic volcanic sediments associated with submarine volcanism. The nature of the formation changed with time, becoming increasingly dominated by basaltic and andesitic lava flows. Some of these formed underwater to become pillowed flows. The seascape, which back then lay in a tropical setting, may have resembled today's volcano-rimmed, earthquake-prone Molucca Sea of central Indonesia.

Remnants of the Tuttle Lake formation exist as a generally east-west band that extends from the lower Glen Alpine Creek drainage west to Susie Lake and Jacks Peak and from Mt. Tallac west to Half Moon Lake and Dicks Peak (and along the ridge north from it). Because peaks, ridges, cliffs, and slopes have developed in this formation, it is very prominent, painting the east-central part of Desolation Wilderness in earth tones. In contrast, the equally colorful Sailor Canyon formation often goes unnoticed, for it exists largely amid talus and vegetation of generally bottom-lands and lower slopes.

Whereas volcanoes developed in this area and produced lava or tephra (ejected material, from fine ash to huge blocks), part of the molten material that fed the volcanoes solidified within them or close to the surface of adjacent bedrock. Magma that produced basaltic lava also solidified to form subsurface gabbro, and magma that produced andesitic lava also solidified to form subsurface diorite. You see quite a lot of these dark, intrusive rocks along Hike 7, first from before Maud Lake and most of the way up to Rockbound Pass, and then from Lake Lois to Lake Schmidell. Likewise, each of the three Velma Lakes (Hike 20) is almost entirely surrounded by diorite or gabbro, as is the floor of the canyon that descends northeast from them to Emerald Bay.

The Sierra's most common intrusive (plutonic) rock is granodiorite, a rock that gives the range its characteristic light-gray color. It and closely related forms (granite, alaskite, quartz monzonite) are often called granitic rocks. During this time of volcanism, some magma cooled to form granitic plutons, and four remain today. These are, from oldest to youngest, Keiths Dome quartz monzonite (area bounded by Ralston Peak, Echo Peak, and Heather Lake), Pyramid Peak granite (crest lands from that peak north to Red Peak), Desolation Valley granodiorite (in its namesake and in upper Rockbound Valley), and Camper Flat granodiorite (Phipps Peak west across Camper Flat to Highland Lake and beyond).

Uplift, Metamorphism, and More Plutonism

The Sierra Nevada finally became a mountain range during the Nevadan orogeny, a compressional "event" that in our area lasted from about 163 to 143 million years ago. During this time, five terranes (pieces of the earth's crust) were individually compressed against and then accreted (attached) to lands west of our area. Each compression probably caused some uplift, and after the last one our area had reached much greater elevations than those of today. Each compression also probably caused some metamorphism of the existing rocks, that is, transforming them through heat and pressure. Sedimentary rocks became metasedimentary ones, and volcanic rocks became metavolcanic ones, and they were both folded and faulted.

Compression can thicken continental crust only to a certain extent before it becomes too heavy to be supported by the underlying plastic, slowly deforming rock. As the underlying rock began to flow, the newly formed Sierra Nevada began to extend apart, and its crust thinned, in part fracturing the existing plutons. This rifting greatly facilitated the upward flow of deep-seated magma, and the range entered a period of voluminous volcanism and plutonism. Large volcanoes developed on the surface, while large bodies of magma just below them solidified to form plutons. The oldest post-orogeny plutons are about 143 to 140 million years old, and on Highway 50 east you drive past their exposed granitic rocks first near the west part of Placerville and then later from about Riverton onward for several miles.

Many of the granitic rocks found in Desolation Wilderness and the lands south of it are considerably younger. Here a second group of plutons developed that are about 100 to 85 million years old. They too once had volcanoes and lava flows above them, but all that has been removed. This is because the magma that produced the granitic plutons produced volcanoes of rhyolite and dacite. These rocks solidified from lava so stiff, viscous, and gas-charged, that violent eruptions often resulted, producing voluminous ash deposits. These were readily eroded and deposited as sediments in the Central Valley. Pasty rhyolite and dacite flows that developed in our area were weathered and eroded over time so that they too no longer exist. Unlike the earlier basalt and andesite flows, these were never metamorphosed into more-resistant rocks.

Development of a Granitic Landscape

The extension that caused voluminous volcanism and plutonism also rifted the crust along faults. The crust immediately east of the wilderness was down-faulted, creating the Truckee—Lake Tahoe depression. (Lake Tahoe formed much later). Other depressions also were created along faults, including the Mono Basin and Owens Valley.

Roughly about 80 million years ago and continuing perhaps for one to several million years, the upper crust of the central Sierra Nevada collapsed, perhaps due to the cessation of plutonism in the range. Apparently the range's upper crust was faulted along a detachment fault, one that separated the brittle upper crust from the ductile, slowly deforming lower crust. With the weight of several miles of thickness removed, the lower crust raised to roughly its present height. Back then, dinosaurs roamed the Sierran lands, until their extinction at 65 million years ago.

The climate during the days of the dinosaurs was tropical, and after their demise it still remained moist and warm until about 33 million years ago, when it began to change toward California's modern summer-dry climates. Under moist and warm climates the sedimentary and volcanic rocks weathered and eroded quite rapidly, and the tops of granitic plutons were exposed in as little as several million years. By 65 million years ago, our area, like most of

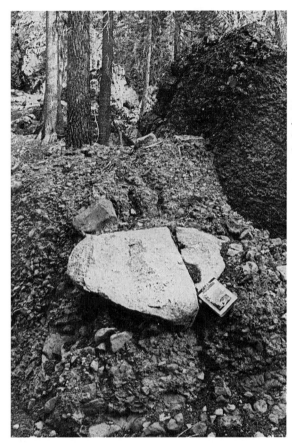

Five-foot long granitic boulder carried in volcanic mudflow

the Sierra Nevada, had become a largely granitic landscape. By 33 million years ago, this landscape had evolved to one extremely similar to today's granitic landscape—indeed, you could have used today's topographic maps.

Volcanism and Burial

The last pulse of uplift rejuvenated erosion, and coarse sediments were deposited in the lower parts of some drainages. The most important locale, geologically speaking, is the South Yuba River drainage in the vicinity of Malakoff Diggins State Historic Park, north of Nevada City. Minor remnants of these prevolcanic auriferous (gold-rich) gravels let us reconstruct the topography that they buried some 50+ million years ago. What they show is that the South Yuba River canyon back then was essentially as deep as it is today. And, as Waldemar Lindgren had stated back in 1911, the range was just as high.

The 33-million-year date, besides marking climate change, marked the beginning of renewed volcanism. At first there were infrequent, if violent, eruptions of rhyolite. With time, however, there were sufficient eruptions to bury the granitic landscape under as much as 1000 feet of rhyolite, as it did in the Plum Creek drainage south of Riverton. As with the prevolcanic gravels, remnants of rhyolite let us reconstruct the topography they buried. One rhyolite remnant, dated at about 26 million years, buries part of a gully cut through granitic bedrock. This lies just outside our area, about 2 miles east-northeast of the Upper Truckee River's Round Lake (no rhyolite has survived in our area). The remnant shows that this gully above Scotts Lake is not the result of relatively recent glacial erosion, but rather that it had already existed at the time of burial.

The rhyolite outbursts lasted until about 20 million years ago, when floods of volcanic lavas, volcanic mudflows, and volcanic sediments, chiefly andesite in composition, began to inundate the range. (Andesitic volcanism actually *began* earlier, by about 26 million years ago, and it overlapped the waning stage of rhyolitic volcanism.) Geographically centered in the Tahoe area, these deposits extend from the Feather River country south to northern Yosemite National Park. They collectively have been called the Mehrten formation, although more recently this has been subdivided into various units. They eventually covered part of our area with as much as 3000 feet of deposits. Even though volcanism was relatively intense the volcanic landscape was usually quiet, for eruptions probably were no more common than those in today's Cascade Range. In our area the andesitic volcanism, like the earlier rhyolitic volcanism, was largely restricted to south of Highway 50. The greatest andesitic volcanism was in the headwaters of the Upper Truckee River, as one sees along Hikes 30-32. In contrast, Desolation Wilderness largely escaped burial by both periods of volcanism, standing high as an island of granitic and metamorphic rock. Where volcanic deposits were expansive, new rivers originated and carved shallow canyons in them, and these took paths quite different from those of the underlying, former rivers. Occasionally a large lava flow would descend one of these shallow canyons, the best example being the 9-million-year-old Table Mountain flow in the Stanislaus River drainage, south of our area. Between 9 and 5 million years ago the largely andesitic volcanism waned, causing erosion to outpace deposition, and the old river canyons were exhumed.

Creation of Lake Tahoe

As was mentioned earlier, the basin that now holds Lake Tahoe began to form late in the days of the dinosaurs. Over tens of millions of years the bedrock of this Truckee—Lake Tahoe fault-formed basin weathered and eroded. By 33 million years ago, when the climate began to evolve toward the modern one, the southern half (Lake Tahoe part) of the basin had topography that closely resembled today's. Freel Peak, to the east of our area, back then was the basin rim's highest peak, as it is today, and it may have towered over 6000 feet above the basin floor.

The lake began to form about 2¼ million years ago when lava erupted in the northern half of the basin, creating a volcanic dam and effectively impounding water south of it. Between 2¼ and 1¼ million years ago there were at least seven major lava flows, which at times dammed the lake as much as 800 feet above its current 6229-foot level. However, the lake's outlet, the Truckee River, continued to erode through successive flows. Faulting accompanied volcanism in the northern half, but apparently not in the southern half. Geologists nevertheless have mapped a major contemporary fault running along the west side of the lake, despite lack of field evidence. In particular, the thick volcanic deposits at the head of the Upper Truckee River drainage should have been displaced, but no fault movement has been found.

Concluding our look into the origin of Lake Tahoe, we might note that the processes which brought about its creation, early faulting and late volcanism, also denied it national park status. That is because some of the volcanic rocks laid down just east of the Lake Tahoe Basin were faulted, the most famous one being the Comstock fault. Along it, silver, gold, and mercury were injected, creating the Comstock Lode. When it was discovered in 1859, a tide of miners flooded the mining area, and waves of others came to the Tahoe area to cash in on the wealth (see Hike 28 for a bit of mining history). The Tahoe forests were raped for mine timbers, buildings, and firewood, while the mountain meadows were desecrated with livestock that helped feed the hungry hordes. In the Lake Tahoe Basin, traffic utilized a growing network of roads, while laden steamers plied Tahoe's easily navigable waters. Desolation Wilderness, in contrast, was largely spared, except for the livestock. There were no minerals to mine, and because glaciers had removed soils, the trees that grew there were too sparse to be lumbered.

Glaciation

As was just stated. Lake Tahoe owes its origin to a vol-canic dam. Back in the nineteenth century, many believed it had originated after glaciers, through powerful erosion, had excavated a deep basin, which then filled with water. Although this long-per-sisting myth has just about died, the equally long-persisting myth of glaciers as major erosive agents is still alive and well. What gla-ciers do best is transport rockfall; in *resistant* bedrock, they erode very little. Glaciers also accelerate the rate of rockfall production (see Hike 4, Pearl Lake: exfoliation), which explains why glacial deposits are both so bouldery and so voluminous.

In the Tahoe area, small glaciers may have appeared spo-radically as early as 15 million years ago. Major glaciation, howev-er, did not begin until about 2 million years ago. Since then the landscape has been appreciably glaciated perhaps four dozen times. During each major glaciation, glaciers advanced over deposits of previous glaciations, eradicating evidence of their existence. The best glacial records lie not in mountain ranges but rather in ocean sediments, which record alternating periods of glaciation and interglaciation (like the one we are in now). In our area there remains evidence from only two glaciations, the Tahoe and the Tioga. The Tahoe existed from about 200,000 to 132,000 years ago, the slightly smaller Tioga from about 28,000 to 13,000 years ago (although some believe that glaciers mostly were gone by as early as 16,000 years ago). There may have been up to three glaciations between these two, but their glaciers were smaller than the Tioga's, hence no direct evidence of them has survived.

From Desolation Wilderness' west-side Crystal Range, Tahoe glaciers coalesced to form an ice sheet that advanced as much as 10 miles downslope, reaching Union Valley Reservoir. An ice cap formed over the southern half of the wilderness, and gla-ciers spilled outward from it in all directions. The largest one flowed north through Rockbound Valley and down the Rubicon River canyon, ending some 30 miles from its source near Mosquito Pass. As such, it rivaled the Tahoe glacier that flowed through Yosemite Valley. At most, some glaciers on the wilderness' east side advanced about a mile or so beyond Lake Tahoe's west and south-west shores, spewing icebergs into the frigid water.

South of the wilderness, glaciers west of the Sierra crest were relatively small. However, just east of it there existed an enor-mous glacier, 20 miles long, which originated at the Roundtop mountain ice cap and spilled northward into the Upper Truckee River drainage and descended to Lake Tahoe. Because the range above the lake's west shore collected most of the precipitation, the one above its east shore lacked sufficient snow and ice to develop glaciers. However, in the Freel Peak area above the south shore, two north-draining glaciers reached lengths of about 4 miles.

Glaciers not only discharged into Lake Tahoe; a few large ones managed to dam it. These glaciers descended east to the north-flowing Truckee River—Lake Tahoe's outlet stream—and blocked its flow. The glacier dams were immense, high enough to raise the lake's level by 600 feet during an early glaciation. But when water pressure became too great, the ice dams broke, sending an inconceivably large wall of water down the Truckee River canyon. During the Tahoe glaciation, one or more glacier dams raised the lake by 90 feet. Consequently, the lake was larger, and it expanded south over the South Lake Tahoe plain and into the lower part of the Upper Truckee River canyon. Lake-bed sediments were deposited in both areas. During the Tioga glaciation, the glaciers were a bit shorter, and apparently no ice dam formed in the Truckee River canyon. Newer research, done in the late 1990s, indicates that major submarine landslides have occurred within the lake, creating tsunamis ("tidal waves"). Therefore, the "inconceivably large walls of water down the Truckee River canyon" could have been from broken ice dams, tsunamis, or both.

When the Tioga glaciers finally retreated into oblivion about 13,000 years ago, they left behind moraines, which are accumulations of material—mostly rockfall—that the glaciers had transported. In the area covered by this book, the Tahoe and Tioga age moraines are most conspicuous about Fallen Leaf Lake (Hike 12), Cascade Lake (Hike 19), and Emerald Bay (Hike 21). There, lateral moraines formed as boulders carried atop the glaciers fell from their sides, accumulating as a veneer on bedrock ridges. By viewing these moraines, which would have been slightly lower than the surfaces of the glaciers responsible for them, one can visualize the length and thickness of the glaciers. The accompanying map—the extent of glaciers during the Tahoe glaciation—is based on such evidence. Note that most of the area lay under glacier ice.

Overall, glaciers did not radically transform the landscape. Glaciers possibly may have been effective erosive agents only in the Upper Truckee River canyon. There the thick volcanic sequence that had buried the canyon, which is composed of volcanic silts, sands, gravels, and a few thin lava flows, are all readily credible. However, most of this sequence would have been removed by the Upper Truckee River in the approximately 10 million years it had to erode before glaciation. When glaciation com-

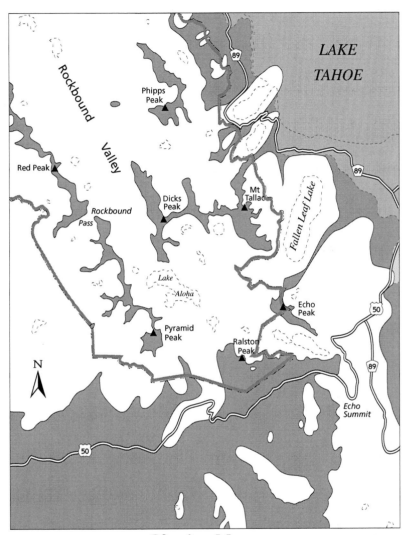

Glacier Map

Author's reconstruction of glaciers in the Fallen Leaf Lake quadrangle, showing their maximum extent during the Tahoe glaciation, which occurred from about 200,000 to 132,000 years ago. Glaciated lands are shown in white, nonglaciated lands in gray. Today's lakes, roads, and wilderness boundary are shown as dashed black lines. The water level of Lake Tahoe back then was up to 90 feet higher, hence its larger size. In Desolation Wilderness only the major peaks and crests stood above glacier ice, but just south of Highway 50 the lands remained largely unglaciated.

menced, the buried granitic surface of the upper drainage may have been largely exhumed or else may have lain under a thin layer of volcanic sediments.

Before glaciation, granitic bedrock locally had undergone considerable weathering, particularly on flat-floored canyon bottoms, where the weathering front penetrated along fractured bedrock. Glaciers removed this weathered bedrock, excavating hollows that then became today's lakes. Had Desolation Wilderness been volcanic rather than granitic, it would have been virtually lakeless. Superficially, Round Lake in the Upper Truckee River drainage (Hike 30) seems to be completely rimmed by such rocks, but closer inspection reveals granitic rocks along its floor and its west shore.

In addition to excavating generally shallow lake basins, glaciers have modified the landscape by accelerating two processes of mass wasting. First, they have caused accelerated rockfall due to pressure release. Large, thick glaciers exist for thousands of years, and their mass applies considerable pressure to the bedrock. When they melt away, which happens rather suddenly, the bedrock becomes depressurized. Slopes and cliffs then undergo accelerated mass wasting, spalling rock slabs that break and accumulate below as talus (which future glaciers will remove). Second, because glaciers produce extremely cold local climates, freeze-and-thaw prying of rocks is also accelerated. This is particularly true at the heads of glaciers, where snowfields today linger long into summer. Conventional wisdom has held that cirques developed as the heads of glaciers plucked away at the adjoining bedrock. However, a bergschrund (the glacier's uppermost crevasse) separates the ice from the wall—plucking cannot occur where there is no contact!

Parts of our area remain almost as pristine and desolate as the day the glaciers left them, for in areas of soil-free bedrock, the granite has weathered only a fraction of an inch in the last 13,000 years. But hardy plants and animals have adapted to this bleak environment. A sparse number of drought-tolerant conifers, shrubs, and wildflowers painstakingly work away at granitic cracks, gradually enlarging their roothold on the land as they change it for their benefit and that of future plants. Animals such as marmots and pikas dwell in talus slopes of granitic rock, stirring up its sterile gravel as they shape their burrows. Their food scraps and feces add nutrients to the gravel, enriching it for plants. Thus plants and animals slowly change the environment to better suit themselves even as the environment is influencing evolutionary changes in them.

Biology

Introduction

To adequately cover Tahoe's plants and animals, their interrelationships, and their influences on—and influences by—the environment is a difficult task if one attempts to do so in only a few pages. You can find a book or two on each Sierran life form and its ecology: on wildflowers, on shrubs, on trees, on birds, on mammals, and so on (see **Recommended Reading and Source Books**). Most amateur naturalists exploring the Tahoe area come to view its wildflowers and birds. For wildflowers, use Niehaus and Ripper's *Field Guide to Pacific States Wildflowers*, which covers a very large area but nevertheless does a good job of identifying the Sierra's common wildflowers. (The common names for wildflowers are based mostly on this guide. Where alternate common names exist, these are mentioned below in parentheses.) If you prefer color photos to botanical keys, try Graf's fairly complete *Plants of the Tahoe Basin*. Its primary drawback (another is a virtually useless index) is that you will have more than 220 pages of photos to pore over, so for the book to be effective, you've got to memorize the photos! A key would be useful, and for that get Weeden's comprehensive *A Sierra Nevada Flora*, which is for those doing serious plant study. Horn's *Sierra Nevada Wildflowers*, which has some species beyond our area, may be better than Graf's book, simply because it has fewer photos to pore over, and these are larger. For serious plant study, lug along the hefty authority, Hickman's *Jepson Manual: Higher Plants of California*. Finally, for a comprehensive introduction to the area's flowers by a competent, vivacious botanist who is obviously enamored by them, get Carville's *Lingering in Tahoe's Wild Gardens*, which not only mentions flowers seen along 30 Tahoe trails, but also gives fascinating details about each. Even if you never hike a trail, simply reading her book will give you quite a thorough education in wildflowers.

If birds interest you, carry the new authoritative book, *The Sibley Guide to Birds*. Also bring along, or study beforehand, Games' *Birds of Yosemite and the East Slope*, which is very fitting for Tahoe species. Arranging birds by habitat, this guide makes the identification of hard-to-view birds an easier task. If you're interested in all aspects of nature, carry Storer and Usinger's *Sierra Nevada Natural History*, which, though dated, is still perhaps the best introduction to the range's plants and animals.

Habitats

When you hike in the mountains—or anywhere, for that matter—you anticipate seeing certain plants and animals in a given habitat. You quickly learn, for example, that junipers don't grow in wet meadows, but corn lilies do. Corn lilies, in turn, don't grow on dry rock slabs, but junipers do. Likewise, you would expect to find garter snakes in wet meadows and western fence lizards on dry rock slabs, but never the reverse. Thus you could group plants and animals by their habitat. In this book this classification is based on the dominant plant or plant types of a habitat, simply because these are the most readily observed life forms. Some habitats are based on topography.

Because animals move, they can be a problem to classify. Birds, for example, typically have a wide—usually seasonal—range, and therefore may be found in many habitats. In the following habitats, a species is mentioned in the one in which a summer visitor is most likely to see it. In addition, only the more prominent and/or diagnostic species are mentioned. The habitats are listed in an approximate order of ascending elevation and decreasing temperature.

1. White-Fir Forest

Most of this book's trails begin in the upper reaches of this habitat, where white fir is yielding to red fir. In our area this community of plants and animals is best expressed along Loon Lake (Hike 1), near the shores of Lake Tahoe (Hikes 21 and 24), Emerald Bay (Hikes 21 and 22), and Fallen Leaf Lake (Hike 12). White fir is the dominant conifer, subordinated by ponderosa pine, but also present, usually on drier, more open terrain, are Jeffrey pine, sugar pine, and incense-cedar.

Of all this book's habitats this is the one most likely to erupt into a raging forest fire. *Natural* fires are definitely associated with it. These fires, if left unchecked, burn stands of mixed conifers about once every 10 years. At this frequency, brush and litter do not accumulate sufficiently to result in a damaging forest fire; only the ground cover is burned over, while the trees remain generally intact. Thus, through small burns, the forest is protected from going up in smoke. Eventually, however, it does, since the trees mature, reach old age, and then begin to die. Abundant dead trees, either fallen or standing as snags, invite a conflagration. Some plants are well adapted to fire, and they rapidly invade in the aftermath. (Logging, landslides, and other disruptive elements also bring about invasions.) A patch of charred white-fir snags is likely

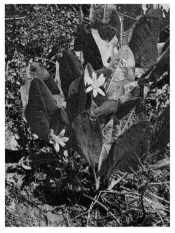

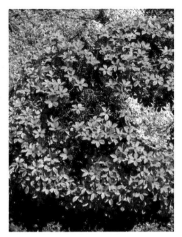

Mule ears   *Spreading phlox*

to be quickly overgrown with tobacco brush, greenleaf manzanita, and, briefly, fireweed.

Many plants and animals found in the white-fir forest are also found in the red-fir forest. Bird watchers, however, might note a few species that definitely prefer the white-fir forest. On its conifers, white-headed woodpeckers punch through the bark to reach wood-boring insects with their long tongues. White-breasted nuthatches descend the trunks head-first, looking for insects in bark crevices, while brown creepers spiral upward in search of same. Higher up in the trees, western tanagers, like Hammond's flycatchers, dart out from the foliage to capture flying insects, though at berry time they're more likely to forage in nearby shrubs. Hermit warblers prefer to stay in the tree foliage, hunting for insects among the branches and needles.

2. Jeffrey Pine—Huckleberry Oak Woodland

In areas of deep soils, white-fir forest grades upward to red-fir forest. Jeffrey pine, a constituent of both, comes into its own where soils become thin, if not downright barren. You may see a healthy specimen seemingly growing right out of a rock slab and, if the day is warm and a gentle breeze blows your way, you may detect the faint butterscotch odor wafted from the furrows of its rusty bark. In spots, shaggy-barked western junipers share the dry, bedrock environment, exuding their own inviting odor. And where volcanic soils abound, fields of mule ears paintbrush may carpet the open-forest slope and lace the air with their distinctive aroma.

But far and away the most common plant associate of the Jeffrey pine is the huckleberry oak. Usually waist-high, this drab, dusty, evergreen oak can form dense, almost impenetrable thickets with occasional Jeffrey pines breaking the monotony. Such thickets are most likely to form on dry, *granitic* slabs and benches. As soils deepen and retain more water, other shrubs appear: greenleaf manzanita, tobacco brush, and bitter cherry. If the soil deepens but remains very dry because it is so gravelly, then snow bush, which because of its spiny tips is also known as mountain whitethorn, joins the huckleberry oaks and Jeffrey pines.

The rocky slabs are seasonally colored with wildflowers. Perhaps the most diagnostic one of this habitat is mountain pride, or Newberry's penstemon. Few wildflowers care to share its masochistic habit, but three that do are spreading phlox, woolly sunflower, and Sierra stonecrop. This dry, rocky environment is ideally suited for western fence lizards, who do push ups to "scare" you away, should you approach too close. The western rattlesnake is another resident, who buzzes at you for the same reason. Chances are you won't see one as you hike the Tahoe landscape. In this habitat the golden-mantled ground squirrel is its main prey.

The sagebrush lizard, a western fence lizard look-alike, prefers dry, gravelly soils. So do a lot of wildflowers. Sunflowers lead the way, with Brewer's daisy, leafy daisy, Anderson's thistle, and yarrow. However, Bridges' penstemon, showy penstemon, Applegate's paintbrush, scarlet gilia (desert trumpet), Leichtlin's

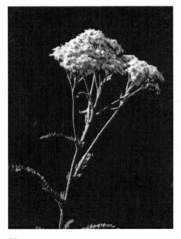

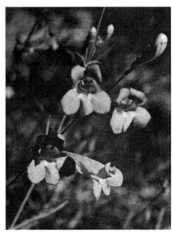

Yarrow   *Showy penstemon*

mariposa lily (tulip), and western wallflower are also bound to catch your attention. In very gravelly soils grow pussy paws, mountain jewel flower (streptanthus, or shieldleaf). Brewer's lupine, nude buckwheat, and sulphur eriogonum (also a buckwheat).

A few Sierran birds definitely prefer this dry, often shrubby environment. Fox sparrows and, to a lesser extent, green-tailed towhees flit about the shrubs, while coveys of

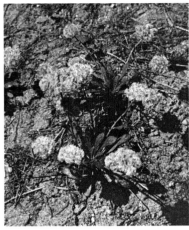

Pussy paws

mountain quail dart about on the ground. On rockier ground, junipers are invaded by Townsend's solitaires when their berries ripen, while Jeffrey pines are occasionally visited by Lewis' woodpeckers.

3. Red-Fir Forest

On the broad, gentle-sloped uplands between the Sierra's mighty river canyons, the red-fir forest can form large, pure stands. In our area, however, canyons and crests characterize the landscape, so the red-fir forest is very heterogeneous. Nevertheless, in its elevation range the red fir accounts for more timberland than lodgepole, Jeffrey, or western white (silver) pine. Most of this book's hikes are up canyons—red-fir country—to lakes, passes, and peaks, so you'll spend most of your *hiking* time in a shady forest. Typically these forested canyons were scoured by glaciers, which then left till ("earth") behind when they retreated. On gentle slopes with adequate soils, red firs do best. On the flat bottom lands, where water content is high, lodgepoles take over, but these mavericks also thrive on steep, gravelly slopes and on rocky outcrops. These two environments normally are the domain of the Jeffrey pine at lower elevations and of the western white pine at higher elevations. Up there, mountain hemlock can locally predominate, particularly where snow cover is thick and long-lasting. This droopy-tipped conifer is equally at home in both the red-fir and subalpine habitats.

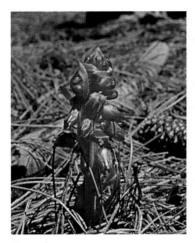

Snow plant

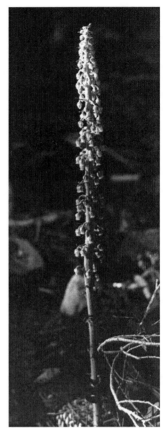

Pinedrops

The red-fir forest gener-
ally is a shady one, and needles
seem to cover the forest floor
more so than bushes or wildflowers. Indeed, in deep-forest shade,
wildflowers are few in both kind
and quantity. However, two plant
families—the heaths and the orchids—thrive in subdued light.
Each family has several species
that can grow even in the absence of light, for these particular
species are saprophytic, that is,
they extract their sustenance from humus—mostly from soil fungi—
rather than from sunlight. Never numerous, the most common
saprophytes are pinedrops, snow plant, spotted coralroot, and
striped coralroot. More exciting, rare finds are sugar stick, fringed
pinesap, and phantom orchid. These saprophytes are easily recognized because, lacking chlorophyll, their stems are not green but
white, yellow, orange, or red. Their green relatives, particularly
dwarf lousewort, white-veined wintergreen, and prince's pine, are
relatively small and are so unobtrusive that hikers rarely notice
them.

Most lowly plants on the *dry* forest floor seek sunny sites.
The most conspicuous of these is the single-stemmed senecio (also
called groundsel or butterweed). Two shrubs common here are
pinemat manzanita—the Sierra's only dwarf manzanita—and bush

chinquapin—with spiny seed capsules and evergreen leaves that are gold on their underside. The great majority of shrubs and wildflowers in the red-fir forest seek *moist*, sunny sites, namely, creeksides. This streamside life is so different from that of the red-fir forest proper that it is described separately under the next category, riparian vegetation.

From a bird's or mammal's viewpoint, there is little to eat on the relatively sterile floor of the shady forest. Hence they usually stay high in the firs and pines, much to the consternation of amateur naturalists. Dropping cones left and right, the diminutive Douglas Squirrel, or chickaree, busily cuts far more cones than it can possibly

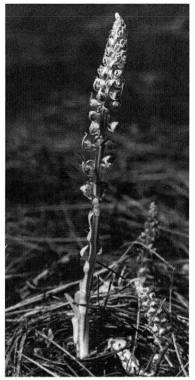

Sugarstick

process, thus aiding conifers in their seed propagation. This talkative squirrel probably evolved in conjunction with montane conifers, specifically, with giant sequoias, which owe a great deal of their existence to the squirrel's seed-dispersing habit. The fossil record indicates that sequoias associated mostly with red firs, whereas today they do so mostly with white firs. The switch occurred because most red firs today grow in glaciated lands, whereas sequoias, which require abundant groundwater, cannot. Consequently, sequoias today grow mostly at the lower elevations of their preglacial altitudinal range.

Keeping squirrels in check, the marten—a member of the weasel family—runs them down, leaping from tree to tree when it's not playing havoc with nesting birds. Look for their dens in rotted-out trunks and snags. Where the forest is more open, golden-mantled ground squirrels and lodgepole chipmunks comb the ground for various seeds, which they store in their rock or log burrows.

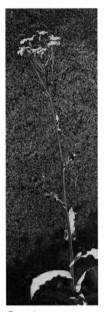
Senecio

Nesting by them among brush is the forest's only ground-dwelling bird, the blue grouse, which in summer has a highly varied diet but in winter limits its consumption mainly to pine and fir needles. This forest is woodpecker country, and you can see at least a half dozen species. One of note, William-son's sapsucker, true to its name goes after sap rather than wood-boring insects, especially preferring the sap of lodgepole and western white pines and, higher up, mountain hem-locks. Combing conifers for bark insects, the red-breasted nuthatch descends the trunk headfirst, then flies to an adjacent one to re-peat the search.

From the lower foliage in dense stands the western wood-peewee shoots out after flying insects, while higher up in the foliage its close cousin, the olive-sided fly-catcher, does the same. Where the forest is more open the dusky flycatcher fills their role. Gleaning insects off branches, twigs, and needles, the tiny golden-crowned kinglet, together with several warblers, peruse the crown. Pruning the tree's seeds and buds are the pine siskin, pine grosbeak, Cassin's finch, and red crossbill—all finches. The red crossbill diverts its energies to eating lodgepole seeds, and its population can drop dramatical-ly if a needleminer moth outbreak decimates these pines. In search of an unwary bird or rodent, the northern goshawk and sharp-shinned hawk patrol the open-forest canopy.

4. Riparian Vegetation

The first three habitats are synonymous with plant com-munities of the same name, for each habitat/community covers a large area. Riparian vegetation differs in that it hugs the creeks that flow down the mountainside, coursing through several plant communities. In our area this habitat is best seen in the red-fir for-est, where the hiker, grown accustomed to the somber tones of browns and muted greens, suddenly comes upon a stream with its sinuous belt of vibrant greens that host a rainbow of colors among its parading wildflowers. Roughly ten species of insects are associ-ated with any wildflower species, and birds take advantage of this abundant harvest.

The shrubs typically are mountain alders and one or more willows. In Tahoe's red-fir belt these are the caudate, dusky, Geyer's, Lemmon's, MacKenzie's, Scouler's, and Sierra willows. American (creek) dogwood, western service-berry, and Sierra currant are fairly common constituents, accompanied in the lower elevations by western azalea and thimbleberry. Mountain ash, in lesser abundance, makes its presence known in September when it produces bright, scarlet berries. About this time the foliage of aspen, black cottonwood, spreading (bitter) dogbane, and bracken fern—all plants thriving on seeps as well as creeks—turn a blazing yellow.

In this moist, usually windless environment, a few wildflowers grow to chest height or more: red-orange-blossomed Sierra tiger (alpine) lily, yellow-blossomed arrowhead butterweed, white-blossomed cow parsnip, and blue-violet-blossomed monkshood and larkspur, both in the buttercup family. Notable waist-high buttercups are the red columbine and the distinctly nonmeadow meadow rue, which is *dioecious*, that is, it has male flowers on one plant, female flowers on another. This is a rare trait for wildflowers. Other wildflowers you're likely to note at streamside are Richardson's geranium, giant red paintbrush, Lewis' monkey flower, and broadleaf lupine, this lupine occurring in a wide variety of environments having abundant soil moisture.

As a rule, conspicuous mammals don't reside among streamside vegetation, although small ones do, particularly the western jumping mouse, vagrant shrew, water shrew, and mountain beaver (aplodontia). The last two readily take to the water. Not a

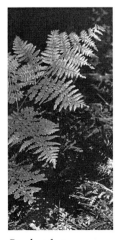 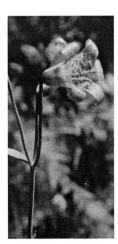 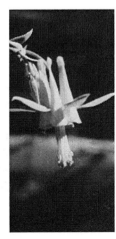

Bracken fern   *Alpine lily*   *Red columbine*

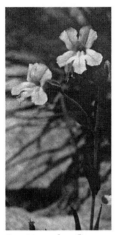
Lewis' monkey flower

beaver, the mountain beaver more closely resembles an overgrown pocket gopher. Beavers once were common in the Sierra Nevada, but over most of their range were trapped into oblivion. Locally they have been reintroduced, and perhaps your best chance of seeing one is at Lily Lake, by the start of Hikes 14-17. Two other sizable species that frequent this habitat are the porcupine and the black bear. The former browses on willows, alders, aspens, and cottonwoods when it's not girdling pines and firs. The latter, which comes in various colors, is most likely to be seen in late season, during berry season.

Some birds find good foraging among streamside vegetation. The red-breasted sapsucker drills horizontal rows of holes on aspens, alders, black cottonwoods, and other trees such as Scouler's willow (check out these willows along Hike 22). Robins and other thrushes compete with bears for berries while a flurry of feathered friends—various vireos, warblers, and wrens—make inroads on insect populations. The bird most adapted to this streamside habitat—indeed, that can't live without it—is the dipper, a drab, chunky bird that actually forages for aquatic insects on the *bottom* of swift streams, competing with rainbow and eastern brook trout.

5. Mountain Lakes

The wilderness traveler usually comes to the mountains for the lakes, to fish them, to swim in them, or just to admire them. In our area lakes and ponds are "pocket-size" habitats dotting the larger red-fir-forest and subalpine-slopes habitats. The lakes usually are bordered by lodgepole and one or more species of willows, and higher up, by mountain hemlocks. Where the soil is damp, mountain spiraea—a rose with clusters of small, pink flowers often grows. And where it is boggy, there may be a host of heaths.

From the plant family that includes drought-resistant manzanitas and sun-shunning saprophytes, the diverse heath family also includes snow- and water-loving huckleberries. This family's red mountain heather and Labrador tea are common shrubs around most of this area's lakes, the "tea" being easily recognized in any season by the turpentine odor from its leaves. If the shore is exceptionally boggy, American laurel (kalmia) may replace these two. At meadow-bound lakes, expect to see Sierra (dwarf) bilberry forming a low, thick mat, and along many lake inlets and outlets—as well as mountain streams—look for knee-high western blueberry. At the highest lakes white heather (cassiope) displays its tiny, white, bell-shaped flowers, while near inlets on the lowest ones (Lake Tahoe and Loon Lake), western azalea produces large, aromatic flowers.

Glaciers scoured the bedrock that underlies today's mountain lakes, so soil around them is often scant and wildflowers few. Generally one does not visit the lakes to study wildflowers, and few, if any, wildflowers are specifically adapted only to shorelines. However, *within* the lower lakes and ponds there are some unique plants, the most conspicuous one being yellow pond lily. You'll find this large-leaved water lily in ponds that are large enough to survive through the dry summer and in shallow parts of warm lakes. Less showy species include bur-reed, pondweed, arrowhead plant (duck potato), and water-starwort. Grasses and sedges, able to grow deeper, often line floors of mountain lakes.

Lakes with abundant shoreline grass and brush are likely to attract mallards and spotted sandpipers, both nesting in such shoreline vegetation. In late summer another water bird, the eared grebe, flies in to browse at these lakes. Pursuing aerial insects, several species of fly-catchers dart out over a lake's shore, while the violet-green swallow swoops across its waters. As evening approaches, bats—particularly the little brown myotis—take over the harvesting chores, occasionally aided by a leaping trout.

And for some visitors, trout are what lakes are all about. Of the approximately seven dozen lakes mentioned in this book, about 70% are stocked with eastern brook trout, 40% with rainbow, 15% with golden or brown, and only 5% with cutthroat. The eastern brook trout does best in high lakes, which is why it is so common in this area. Furthermore, it can spawn in lakes, whereas the others typically need streams.

Because most backpackers camp at lakes, black bears *occasionally* are attracted to them. If you are worried about losing your food, you could bearbag it (see illustration). If you are not familiar with this method, see the bearbagging section in Winnett and Findling's *Backpacking Basics*. Since the mid-'90s, another option has been available: bear-resistant food canisters. These are bulky, heavy, and quite expensive, but they work well and also protect against rodents. You can compensate for their extra weight by wearing *backpacking* (not *beach*) sandals, which reduce your hiking effort.

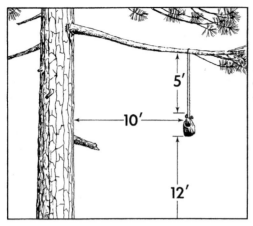

Recommended minimum distance for bearbagging on a tree branch

5'

10'

12'

6. Mountain Meadows

Often meadows go hand in hand with lakes, though either can exist without the other. There has been a long-standing view that meadows are just former lakes that have been completely filled in with sediments. Given enough time, this will happen, but Tahoe's mountain lakes have existed only about 14,000 years, and in that "short" time most have received only about 5 to 20 feet of sediment. In all probability, today's mountain meadows never were lakes. Likewise, given enough time, forests supposedly supplant meadows through a slow process of invasion by water-loving pioneer species, such as the lodgepole pine. But in reality, there is a seesaw battle between forest and meadow, and in times of wetter climate, a meadow will expand at the expense of its encroaching forest.

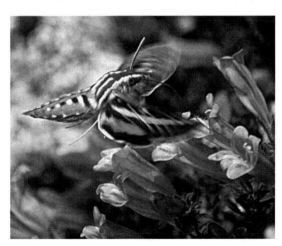

Sphinx moth and penstemons

Cattle-free meadows abound with wildflowers, cattle-trodden ones do not. Cattle in the Tahoe area go back to mining days, when they were brought to the mountain meadows to provide nearby mining settlements with milk, cheese, and meat, particularly after most of the native game had been overhunted. At present cattle are brought in to graze *western* Desolation Wilderness in August and September, and a similar grazing schedule exists in this area's mountain meadows outside the wilderness. You can avoid the cattle by hiking to these areas in early or mid-July, but my God, the mosquitoes! Hordes of them. And their numbers unfortunately peak just when wildflowers usually are at

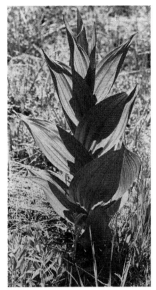

Corn lily

their best. But while you may curse these needling females (males don't suck blood), you should bear in mind—as you try to identify or appreciate the meadow's wildflowers—that many of the small-flowered species may in part rely on mosquitoes for propagation. Lungworts and rein orchids are definitely known to be mosquito-pollinated.

Thumbnail-size Pacific tree frogs aid a number of birds in cutting down the mosquito population: white-throated swifts, violet-green swallows, and cliff swallows soar and dive overhead while dusky flycatchers and western wood-peewees sally forth from trees and shrubs in and about the meadow. Lincoln's sparrows, dark-eyed juncos, and Brewer's blackbirds search wet meadows for seeds as well as insects, joined in drier meadows by chipping sparrows. Aiding bees, flies, beetles, and mosquitoes in pollinating a meadow's flowers are rufous hummingbirds, which sometimes compete with large sphynx moths, particularly for long-tubed flowers such as penstemons, paintbrushes, and monkey flowers, all belonging to the figwort, or snapdragon, family.

Meadowland is rodent land, and an amazingly large population of mice, voles, and shrews inhabit and harvest it. In drier parts of meadows Belding ground squirrels join in the harvest as do pocket gophers and broadfooted moles. All three burrow underground, but do not compete with one another. The ground squirrel eats surface vegetation, the pocket gopher mostly roots, tubers, and bulbs, and the mole mostly subsurface invertebrates. The pocket gopher in particular can create quite an extensive tunnel system, and in a mountain meadow a population can churn up tons of soil each year. The others do so to a lesser degree. This churning has its benefits, for it leads to the development of a richer, better aerated soil, which in turn can benefit the meadow's flora.

In meadows northern harriers (marsh hawks) and American kestrels (sparrow hawks) prey on numerous meadowland birds and mammals, while their larger relatives, the red-tailed hawks, soar overhead in search of a hapless rodent. At dusk, great horned owls emerge from the forest's edge for the meadowland's "graveyard" rodent patrol. On the ground two closely related species, the weasel and the ermine, probably are the rodents' major predators.

The beauty of the wildflowers is what calls some to mountain meadows. A tall plant of wet meadows is the corn lily, named for its cornlike leaves. A rarer monocot is swamp onion, with rosy flowers, which lives up to its name by inhabiting the wettest meadows. In contrast, western blue flag, an iris, prefers drier ground. The great bulk of the meadow's monocots—its grasses and sedges—are not showy.

Many dicots vie for your attention—as well as that of pollinating insects. The sunflower family, whose "flowers" are actually flower heads composed of numerous closely packed flowers, have a number of entries. Two of the showier, yellow-flowered ones are meadow goldenrod and Bigelow's sneezeweed, both common in the

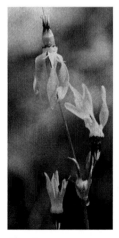

Shooting star

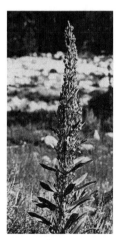

Deer's tongue

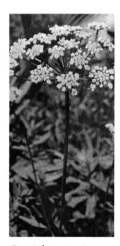

Gray's ligusticum

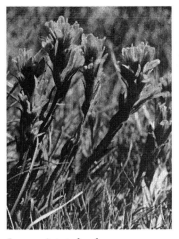

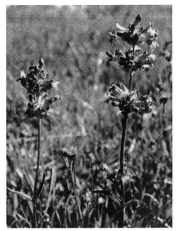

Lemmon's paintbrush   *Whorled penstemons*

lower meadows. Higher up are two look-alikes, the western mountain aster and the wandering daisy (daisy fleabane), both with lavender *ray* flowers surrounding yellow *disk* flowers. Possessing only yellow ray flowers is the nodding microseris, which closely resembles the dandelions commonly found in lawns.

In the rose family, cinquefoils are perhaps the most conspicuous meadow plants. Look for Brewer's, slender, and sticky cinquefoils along meadow edges and damp slopes. Similar-looking flowers, the buttercups, lack bracts beneath the flower's sepals. The commonest buttercup in Sierran meadows appears to be the water plantain buttercup, named for its plantainlike leaves.

Where you find corn lily, you'll usually find Jeffrey's shooting star, a nodding, lavender-petaled flower that turns upright after it's been pollinated. Near it you may see three gentians. The monument plant (deer's tongue, green gentian) grows to head height. Its two distant relatives, the many-flowered explorer's gentian and the single-flowered hiker's gentian, are so short they are often lost among the other vegetation. In contrast, the bistort, a buckwheat, sends its white, flower-packed puffballs up to knee height or more.

The carrot, or parsley, family offers its white-blossomed Gray's ligusticum. Brewer's angelica, and Parish's yampah for your inspection. Members of this family have their flower heads arranged like an umbrella, hence the old (now abandoned) family name Umbelliferae. Taproots and leaves of this family can be either nutritious *or* deadly, so don't experiment.

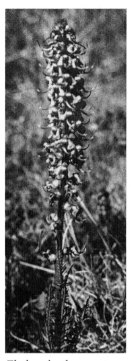
Elephant heads

Finally, the figwort family offers its typically showy assemblage of paintbrushes, penstemons, and monkey flowers. Notable species are Lemmon's and Peirson's paintbrushes, meadow and Sierra penstemon (both of them "whorled" penstemons), and common (seep-spring) monkey flower. In higher meadows that border on bogs, look for the delicate, purple blossoms of aptly named elephant heads and little elephant heads. In meadows where paintbrush is common, it often codominates with lupines which, though in the pea family, definitely are not edible. Large-leaved (blue-pod, marsh, superb) lupine, growing to 4 feet high, is a species common both in wet meadows and along creeksides.

7. Subalpine Slopes

In some books you'll find this habitat, which is also a plant community, identified as "subalpine forest." Forest it is not. Its tree cover is quite discontinuous and, as you approach its upper-elevation limit, you'll note that trees often become quite sparse. All of the preceding habitats listed in this chapter can be subdivided into smaller ecological units, and the subalpine-slopes habitat is no exception. Because it is relatively open, you can stand in one spot and observe this habitat's four major subdivisions: forest, meadow, rock, and gravel.

One such spot is on the Ralston Peak Trail (Hike 9), where the trail tops out on a "generally open ridge," and you then begin a 0.6- mile climb eastward to the peak's summit. This spot, at about 8870 feet elevation, is in the low-to-mid range of the subalpine-slopes habitat. You stand by a cluster of mountain hemlocks, while just east of it you see your hiking route up an open "forest" of lodgepole and whitebark pines. The whitebark pines, which are the timberline species in the Tahoe area, become more numerous as you climb eastward. Where the microclimate is extremely harsh, these trees may be dwarfed and contorted, in short, *krummholtz* (literally, "crooked wood"). Just north of and

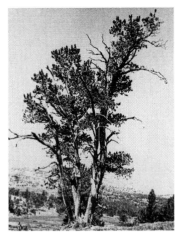

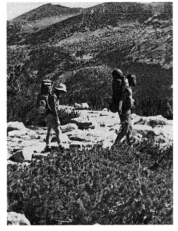

Whitebark pine tree   *Krummholtz whitebark pine*

below you lies a small subalpine meadow that is, like others of its elevation, almost always soggy. Your showiest subalpine wildflowers are most likely to grow in such an environment. The meadow is bordered on the northeast by granitic bedrock, the logical environment in the subalpine zone in which to look for ferns. Three to look for here and at other damp, dirt-filled cracks among *granitic* bedrock are alpine lady fern, rock-brake (parsley fern), and brittle fern. The slope on the south side of the soggy meadow is mantled with granite-derived gravel. On this very loose slope, nothing grows, for it is usually covered by an almost permanent snowfield. This gravel is derived from the ridge on which you start your summit hike. Being unglaciated, it has been exposed to the elements far longer than any glaciated terrain, so its *granitic* bedrock has had more than ample time to decompose to loosely packed gravel. Water retention is poor in such nutrient-poor soils, and the wildflowers that choose such a harsh environment must grow while adjacent snowfields are melting and/or utilize water-conserving techniques.

In the preceding paragraph granitic rocks have been emphasized because metamorphic rocks produce richer soils. This is in part because metamorphic bedrock fractures into smaller pieces than granitic bedrock does, creating a greater water-storage capacity for plants. Furthermore, this rock is much richer in dark minerals, so it yields a more nutrient-rich soil. And, being darker in color than their granitic counterparts, metamorphic-derived soils absorb more heat—very important to plants at these higher,

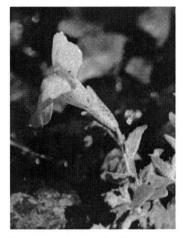 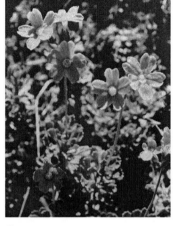

Large mountain monkey flower   *Sierra primroses*

cooler elevations. But volcanic bedrock surpasses all others in soil formation. The dark, nutrient-rich rock breaks down into very fine, clay-rich particles that not only hold a lot of water in their interstitial spaces, but also may absorb water into their clay structure. (Trails across *wet* volcanic soil or decomposed rock are quite slippery!) Thus the best wildflower gardens should grow in volcanic soils, which are found in abundance on and below the Sierra crest below Echo Summit and Carson Pass (particularly along Hikes 30-32). Unfortunately, the gardens may be sub-optimal, due to past cattle grazing.

In the subalpine-slopes habitat, wildflowers seem to do best in seeps, which are miniature meadows usually watered by a nearby snow patch. In some you may see a nearly homogeneous bed of a particular wildflower. For instance, the mountain helenium, a sunflower poisonous to cattle, may locally paint an otherwise drab hillside yellow with its hundreds of yellow-blossomed plants. On a smaller scale, common monkey flowers and mountain monkey flowers locally dab the landscape a vibrant yellow. And what amateur botanist wouldn't be thrilled to find—perhaps along with ferns—a band of Sierra primroses or a cluster of rockfringes, both adding pink to an icy, gray environment? This high, cold, wet environment is saxifrage country. Up here you'll find alumroot, mitrewort, grass-of-parnassus, gooseberry, currant—all in the saxifrage family—plus a number of true saxifrages, particularly Sierra and bud saxifrage. These two thumb-size plants can be found with a

very notable subalpine but-
tercup-family member, the
marsh marigold.

While water lasts
on gravel slopes, yellow
Sierra wallflowers can put
on quite a show, comple-
mented by dwarf (Lobb's
and Lyall's) lupine, and at
times by alpine paintbrush.
As gravel gives way to broken rock, leptodactylon
and spreading phlox assert
their presence, accompa-
nied by sunflowers such as
silky and green-leaved rail-
lardellas and cut-leaved
and Sierra daisies. Several
shrubs gravitate toward this hostile
environment but, lacking flowers
most of the time, they are often
hard for the novice to identify. To
narrow your choices, the author
suggests you read up on the vegetation characteristics of bush cinque-
foil, ocean spray, timberline sagebrush, and the several species of
similar looking rabbitbrush and
goldenbush. Where loose rock
gives way to dry, sunny bedrock,
look for Davidson's penstemon,

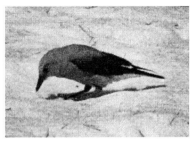

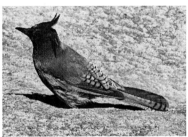

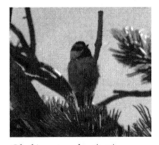

Clark's nutcracker (top)
Steller's jay (middle)
Mountain chickadee (bottom)

which, with its long-tubed, purple blossoms, is far more conspicuous than several species of eriogonums (buckwheats).

The plants growing in gravelly or rocky areas are harvest-
ed by alpine chipmunks, pikas, yellow-bellied marmots, and golden-mantled ground squirrels. Only the first two are true high-ele-
vation species, the two others extending their range down as low
as 6000 feet. All four may look for handouts on popular peaks such
as Tallac and Ralston.

The most noticeable subalpine bird is the Clark's nutcracker, a large, grayish, noisy relative of the Steller's jay, found
below in open conifer forests. The nutcracker typically feeds on
seeds of the whitebark and lodgepole pines, though it may also feed

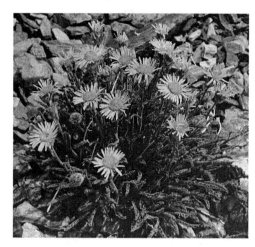

Alpine gold

on those of mountain hemlock and western white pine. Other birds commonly seen up in the subalpine environments—as well as in lower ones— are robin, junco, mountain chickadee, and chipping and white-crowned sparrows. Cassin's finch eats conifer buds, seeds, and berries, as does its red-fir-belt cousin, the pine grosbeak, whose feeding habits in turn are similar to those of a lower-elevation relative, the evening grosbeak. In the highest reaches of the subalpine zone, the mountain bluebird flutters about in search of aerial and ground insects.

8. Alpine

Consider yourself in the alpine habitat if you see a rosy finch; it seems to prefer only the highest summits. The summits of Mt. Tallac, Ralston Peak, and Echo Peak are marginal alpine habitats. Trailless Pyramid Peak, less than a stone's throw below the 10,000-foot level, is a better candidate. For a truly alpine experience in the Tahoe area you'll have to climb to about 2 miles high, conquering Mt. Rose (10,776) at the area's north end, Freel Peak (10,881) at its south end, or Stevens and Red Lake peaks (10,059 and 10,061), above the Upper Truckee River basin. The mustard and sunflower families seem to have a disproportionate number of alpine species. The former boasts several species of rock cress and draba, while the latter has an even greater assortment. Perhaps the most beautiful sunflower is alpine gold, growing on or near these peaks' summits. Finally, showy polemonium, a member of the phlox family, adds specks of pale-blue to mountaintops, especially on Mt. Tallac. Drop your pack and take time, if weather permits, to get acquainted with this habitat's miniature, tenacious flora.

Chapter 4

Thirty-Two
Hikes

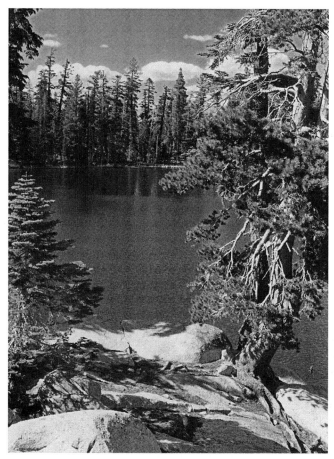

Lost Lake

Loon Lake Trail

HIKE 1

Maps

2 and 3

Distances

4.1 miles to Pleasant Campground by Loon Lake

4.5 miles to Spider Lake

5.3 miles to Lake Winifred

6.1 miles to Buck Island Lake

6.7 miles to Rockbound Lake

8.2 miles to Fox Lake

8.3 miles to Rubicon Reservoir

11.7 miles to AAA Camp

13.5 miles to McConnell Lake (4-Q Lakes) Trail

13.6 miles to Camper Flat

13.8 miles to Blakely (Lake Schmidell) Trail

Directions to trailhead

If you plan to enter the wilderness (Rockbound Lake and beyond), be sure to get a wilderness permit (see Chapter 2's section on wilderness permits). The best place to get one is at the Eldorado National Forest Information Center, on Camino Heights Drive about 5 miles east of Placerville. From this center continue 17 miles east up Highway 50 to its bridge across the South Fork American River and in 100 yards reach the Crystal Basin Recreation Area turnoff, Ice House Road, on your left. (Westbound drivers: this junction is about 27 miles west from Echo Summit.)

Your road, paved all the way to the trailhead, climbs 9 miles to Ice House Resort. Farther north, your Forest Route 3 passes the Crystal Basin Ranger Station as well as spur roads to Union Valley Reservoir's campgrounds. After a 13-mile winding course from the resort you reach the Loon Lake Road, branching right. Signed Forest Route 3, you take it 4½ miles to a fork. Left, a road goes 3¼ miles over to Loon Lake's far dam. You branch right and go 0.4 mile to an entrance to a horse camp, then just past it, branch right. You curve briefly to reach a third branch. Older campsites lie along the road branching left. You keep right, past newer camp-sites, briefly to a trailhead parking lot at road's end.

Introduction

For relatively easy hiking in Desolation Wilderness, take this route. The 13.7-mile one-way distance has only minor ups and downs and, if you hike to its end, you'll gain only 800 feet in ele-vation. In late June and early July, when most of the Desolation Wilderness lakes are still frozen or just thawing, the seven lakes along this route provide good fishing and brisk swimming.

Route description

Beginning at the far end of the trailhead parking lot, the Loon Lake Trail goes but 60 yards to a junction with a trail from the horse camp. Your trail now goes 160 yards to another junction, this time with a 150-yard-long feeder trail ascending northeast from the far end of the old-campsites section of the multi-part Loon Lake Campground. Ahead, the trail soon parallels the lake's visible shoreline, usually keeping about 100 yards distant. About ½ mile beyond the campground the trail almost touches the lake, and soon traverses around a 15-foot-high boulder, an erratic transport-ed here by the last glacier. This boulder is considerably larger than others nearby, though hardly a 1000-ton mega-erratic.

Beyond these boulders the trail soon bends east-northeast for a mile-long, fir-and-pine-shaded traverse that passes a seasonal creeklet soon after your first glimpse of Brown Mountain. This stands about ½ mile southeast, and it may be the remnants of a small, basaltic volcano. Glaciers removed its looser rock, and topped it at least once, as evidenced by the granitic rocks left behind on its summit.

About 2½ miles from the trailhead we climb to a ridge, whose northwest extension almost divides the lake in two. Before 1967, when the new dam was completed, this ridge separated Pleasant Lake from Loon Lake. As we make an eastward traverse, we see possible brushy descent routes to the shoreline, these in the direction of bald-topped Guide Peak, which juts prominently sky-ward behind the lake. Continuing eastward, one has good views

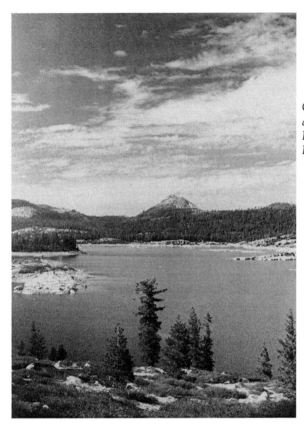

Guide Peak rises above Loon Lake's "Pleasant Lake" arm

ahead toward a saddle, between two unnamed peaks, in which lies Hidden Lake.

After the traverse we momentarily turn south into a gully to cross its creek, then turn north and gradually descend to an abandoned road that descends to the east arm of Loon Lake. We make a short climb north up this closed road to a roadcut blasted out of bedrock, exposing a thick, light-colored vein, or dike. From it we can look southwest across the lake to its dam and the hills beyond. At the shoreline below us is a hidden cove visited by boaters. In ¼ mile our road reaches a gully and begins a moderate climb west. Here you can take a 0.4-mile spur trail to **Pleasant Campground**. Just before one reaches the actual campground, one has to leave the gully and cross northwest over a low ridge. The campground, which has tables, stoves, and an outhouse, is primarily for boaters. There is no fee for this campground, and no piped water. Consider a day visit to this area to fish or swim along the shore.

Back on the closed road again, we climb northwest to a ridge, then follow it east up to a broad saddle, leaving views of the Loon Lake terrain for those of the gentle Sierra crest. Northeast of and not far below the trail lies a linear, seasonal, lily-pad pond. About 100 yards beyond it you should see the western arm of **Spider Lake**, to which you could descend. Campsites lie about the sprawling lake, and don't be content with the first vacant one you spy. About ¼ mile farther southeast on our road you reach a low ridge on which you could also descend directly to near the lake's shallow south arm. This route, one of several possible, begins just as you reach a long, straight stretch of road. Just before this route junction you could have begun a cross-country route southwest ½ mile up relatively open slopes to the Hidden Lake saddle. Onward, we walk about 0.4 mile on our road, first gently down, then gently up to a second broad saddle. From it an easy ⅓-mile cross-country jaunt southwest takes one over a low ridge and down to campsites beside tranquil **Lake Winifred**. For real seclusion, try visiting one of the lakelets or ponds lying south of this lake.

Most hikers will instead continue along the road, which from the broad saddle makes a long, steady, rocky one-mile descent southeast, crossing a seasonal, cascading creek just before reaching a curve east. Along that short curve is a trail intersection, which can be easily missed if unsigned. In 70 yards the road reaches shallow, rocky **Buck Island Lake** and then climbs ¼ mile southeast back up to the trail (which also goes the same distance to end at the road). In late summer the lake's level can be low and its shoreline desolate. Little water flows from its dammed outlet; rather, the water flows through a tunnel down to Loon Lake, which, like Rockbound and Rubicon reservoirs upstream, is part of Sacramento's water supply system. After Labor Day, Loon Lake loses much of its water, its waterline dropping 30-35 feet by early October. From the trail intersection just above Buck Island Lake the northbound trail goes ½ mile to the lake's dam and just beyond it to the Wentworth Jeep Trail, which, after 1½ miles, approaches the north shore of Spider Lake. Past off-highway vehicles have so impacted parts of this jeep trail that in many places it has been eroded down to bedrock.

If camping at Buck Island Lake looks unappealing when you visit it, due to OHVers, then head into the nearby wilderness. From the trail's end at the road at a bend just above the lake's south shore, take the closed road east, which quickly climbs into Desolation Wilderness and soon traverses over to nearby **Rockbound Lake**. With the addition of a low dam, this lake has been deepened, making it quite appealing before the water drops in late sum-

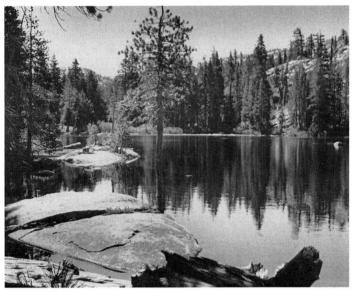

Lake Winifred

mer. As your road curves southeast above this lake, look for small campsites under the sparse tree cover by its south shore.

Near the lake's inlet the road dips into forest cover to quickly reach Highland Lake creek, which has an adjacent campsite. Generally you can rock-hop this wide, attractive creek, then you continue on the road but 180 yards, to where it is blocked off. On your right is a tortuous trail, which you take for 0.3 mile before rejoining the road. This trail segment exists to bypass the "new Rubicon River," up to 15 yards wide, which seasonally gushes from the lower end of a tunnel draining Rubicon Reservoir. On the road you climb about 110 yards to a saddle overlooking **Fox Lake**, which lies 250 yards to the north. From here, competent hikers can strike south, quickly attaining a broad ridge, eventually leaving it to parallel Highland Lake's creek up to the Highland Lake Trail, and then taking that up to the lake (last paragraph of Hike 7).

As your road starts down from the saddle, you can leave the road and make a quick, fairly easy cross-country descent to this tempting lake. On a small island—a peninsula in late summer—several lodgepoles grow beside two large, dark erratics, which are boulders left behind by the last glacier to descend this canyon. Glacial striations mark the direction of its flow.

From the saddle the road descends ¼ mile to a trail junction above the northwest lobe of Rubicon Reservoir. Now on the

Rubicon River Trail we momentarily cross above the reservoir's ¼-mile-long outlet tunnel, then meander south, paralleling the west shore of shallow **Rubicon Reservoir**, which turns into an unattractive mud-and-boulder flat late in summer. We leave this reservoir as the trail curves east, then climb ¼ mile up to two stagnant ponds on a large bench. After a momentary descent the trail climbs mile south to a ford of wide, shallow Rubicon River. To keep your feet dry, try boulder-hopping it about 100 yards downstream.

If you'd like to visit Lake Zitella, you can take a cross-country shortcut up to it. Rather than ford the Rubicon, climb more or less south-southwest up slopes. Half way up, you'll reach a forest on a flat bench and a brushy, short, steep escarpment, which can be climbed unroped (*use caution!*) by several routes. Above, you'll find hiking relatively easy if you stay 100-200 yards from the creek rather than keeping close to it. Cross the creek just below the obvious bench that holds the unseen lake.

Those staying on the trail cross the Rubicon and then start south along low-angle exfoliation slabs, in 300 yards reaching a long, shallow river pool. Just past it you nearly touch the river again, then soon curve east for a ⅓-mile climb upriver to a lodgepole flat, abounding with bracken ferns. Curving across the flat, the trail goes to nearby Phipps Creek, crossing it at the south end of a shallow, wide pool. Now, in a ¼-mile segment, the trail makes a brief, steep climb, then winds south to where ducks mark a 200-yard traverse west to lodgepole-shaded "**AAA Camp**," perched on a bench above the Rubicon. By it the river cascades into a 10-foot-deep pool—brisk, but excellent for diving, cooling off, or just frolicking.

With the Camper Flat area as this hike's goal, we wind southward from the AAA Camp junction, first across the back of a broad, glacially polished ridge, then along the base of its east slopes. Along this undulating stretch a master joint (major fracture in bedrock) lies about 100 yards east of the trail. About ½ mile past the junction you climb southwest to a crest saddle, then drop along a somewhat brushy gully to the nearby river. For ⅓ mile you parallel it up-canyon, noting several large, shallow pools. At a lodgepole thicket where the river bends, you ford it or possibly log-cross it. In this area the trail may be hard to find if hikers have been striking paths up and down the river looking for a dry crossing. If you're on the right track, which starts southeast, you'll reach the north edge of a stagnant pond in about 80 yards. Just ¼ mile past it the trail reaches the Rubicon. Following it gently up-canyon, you pass two of its large, emerald-green pools, the second one at the base of a small cascade. Optimal swimming (still brisk!) is late afternoons in August.

After a few minutes' walk past the second pool, you meet the **McConnell Lake Trail**. If you've got a couple of days to spare, you might make the 4-Q, Horseshoe, McConnell, Leland, Schmidell lakes loop and perhaps even take in Lake Zitella and Highland Lake. All these lakes, which are usually mosquito-ridden and chilly before early August, are described in Hike 7.

Just 70 yards past the McConnell Lake Trail our trail meets Lake Schmidell creek. If it is too high and wide to jump across, look for a log crossing. Past its east bank we slog through a damp meadow, usually very alive with vibrant wildflowers and pesky mosquitoes, then arrive at a spacious campsite at **Camper Flat**. Here you'll find a good, if shallow, Rubicon River swimming hole that tempts you to linger. Shortly beyond this area you'll note a spur trail going west a few yards to a cold, seeping, rust-stained mineral spring. In 70 more level yards you meet the **Blakely Trail**, this hike's end. From here you can travel southwest up to Lake Schmidell (Hike 7), south up-canyon to Lake Aloha (Hike 10), or east up to the Velma Lakes (Hike 20). This last option begins from another trail junction 100 yards south of the Blakely Trail. No camping is allowed along this 100-yard stretch or along a 100-yard stretch south of that junction.

Lyons Creek Trail
HIKE 2

Maps

5

Distances

3.3 miles to Bloodsucker Lake

4.9 miles to Lake Sylvia

5.0 miles to Lyons Lake

Directions to trailhead

If you plan to enter the wilderness (i.e., visit the two lakes), be sure to get a wilderness permit (see Chapter 2's section on wilderness permits). Get one at the Eldorado National Forest Information Center, about 5 miles east of Placerville. From this center continue 26 miles east up Highway 50 to Kyburz, your last stop for food and gas and, after 5 more miles, reach Wrights Lake Road (Forest Route 4), on your left. (The Wrights Lake Road junction is about 13 miles west from Echo Summit, and is easily missed. It is about 4 miles west beyond Strawberry Lodge.) Drive 4.1 miles up this road to an obvious road that branches right only 150 yards before Lyons Creek. There is room on it for about 15 vehicles. Day users can *usually* get a wilderness permit at either the Rockbound trailhead (Hike 4) or the Twin Lakes trailhead (Hike 5).

Introduction

The several meadows along this trail will reward wildflower lovers, while at least three sets of creek pools will please others. However, the main attractions are two subalpine lakes, which by early August can be suitable for swimming. Mountaineers can use either lake as a base camp to ascend three of the wilderness' loftiest summits.

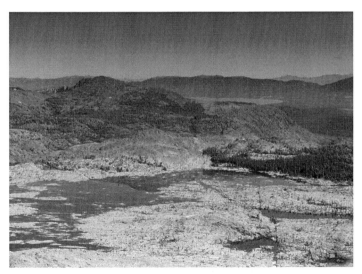

A Pyramid Peak panorama of Desolation Valley

Route description

From the parking area we immediately pass a gate and walk almost 0.4 mile along a closed road to its end. From its southeast side the Lyons Creek Trail climbs gently eastward. Where the trail almost touches the creek, a short spur goes over to a set of shallow pools among granitic slabs. We then pass many seasonal tributaries, as well as several meadows, before reaching the site of Lyons at the edge of another meadow, which like the others presents the best wildflowers in July. Just as our trail climbs east to leave this meadow, the Bloodsucker Lake Trail cuts west-northwest to Lyons Creek, which is boulder-hopped. This way up to **Bloodsucker Lake** is 1.5 miles longer than is Hike 3. See that hike's last paragraph for a brief description (in reverse) of the ascent northwest.

About 1.4 miles past the Bloodsucker Lake Trail, from just beyond the Desolation Wilderness border, you can take a short spur northwest to a second set of slab pools, deeper than those near the trailhead. Then, climbing up open, granitic slopes, you have your first view of Pyramid Peak, and you reach a third set of pools just before crossing lodgepole-lined Lyons Creek. After 200 yards east from the crossing, you reach a junction. The branch east quickly reaches and then traverses a 50-yard-long swath of creeks, which is usually boggy through mid-July, then climbs ¼ mile to shallow, placid, trout-inhabited **Lake Sylvia**. Although this 8050-foot lake lacks impressive views like those found along the Lyons Creek Trail, it does have some large, good campsites, under a canopy of shady conifers, and in early August a swim can be fairly warm. This locale is a good base camp for a climb up Pyramid Peak, which towers almost 2000 feet above the lake. To reach it, first scramble up to a shallow notch above the lake. This stretch can pose problems due to some loose rocks and, in early season, ice and snow. The rest of the climb is obvious. Summit views, however, are somewhat disappointing since Lake Tahoe is largely hidden from view.

Back at the junction east of Lyons Creek, the left fork climbs north steeply up an open granite slope, affording us views of the often snowbound lower northwest face of Pyramid Peak. The steep ascent ends quickly, and we reach scattered hemlocks near a forebay, which is 3 feet lower than dammed 8380-foot **Lyons Lake**. Small, minimal campsites lie about the lake; Lake Sylvia's sites definitely are better. (Mountaineers may find it necessary to make a base camp at either lake, but to lessen human impact, most visitors should day hike to them.) Like Lake Sylvia, Lyons Lake is fringed with red mountain heather and Labrador tea. Conifers, however, are much more scarce, and the setting is stark and different from that at Sylvia. For experienced mountaineers Lyons Lake is a good base camp for the twin summits of Mts. Price and Agassiz. Both harbor alpine wildflowers, although mountaineering botanists rarely visit their summits.

Bloodsucker Lake Trail

HIKE 3

Maps
5

Distances
1.8 miles to Bloodsucker Lake
5.9 miles to Lake Sylvia
6.2 miles to Lyons Lake

Directions to trailhead

As for the previous hike take Highway 50 to Wrights Lake Road, which begins 36 miles from Highway 49 in Placerville and 13 miles from Echo Summit. Drive 8.0 miles up this road to a trailhead parking area, on your right, reached just 0.2 mile before the Wrights Lake Information Kiosk. Park at the south end of the parking loop.

Introduction

For those who have seen leeches only in the movies, this hike is an eye-opener. It is also an alternate approach to upper Lyons Creek, Lyons Lake, and Lake Sylvia.

Route description

From the Wrights Lake Horse Camp at the south end of the parking loop, begin south on a short trail segment. After 0.1

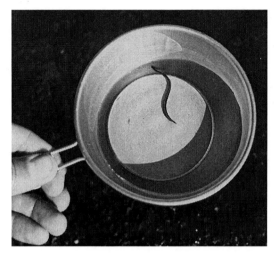

A Bloodsucker Lake leech

mile the trail angles left and drops to a nearby boulder hop of Wrights Lake's South Fork Silver Creek. The trail starts down the creek's east bank, then veers up to a blocked-off road atop a low crest—a moraine. Deposits such as this one allow us to map the former extent of glaciers. From here past glaciers descended several miles southwest to near the east end of Ice House Reservoir.

From the low crest, start east on the closed road, hiking ¼ mile to where it starts a moderate climb. Here on your right is a trail, which in almost 0.7 mile first crosses several streams and then climbs to the Bloodsucker Lake Trail. This trail goes northeast to the lake in just under ½ mile. You, however, keep to the closed road, climbing ¼ mile to cross Secret Lake's outlet creek, and 0.4 mile later reach a switchback on a ridge, just above Bloodsucker Lake's outlet creek. In another ¼ mile your route levels, crosses that creek, and meets the Bloodsucker Lake Trail, described below. Just ahead on the road is knee-deep **Bloodsucker Lake**, with tainted water.

Blue Mountain, with the Crystal Range as a backdrop, adds to the scenic beauty of the lake, but its main attractions are the bloodsuckers—yes, leeches—up to 3 inches long. (You may have to stir the water with your hand to find them.) It seems that the only aquatic species that could serve as hosts for these leeches are yellow-legged frogs, of which there are many. In the absence of frogs, however, the leeches could survive on many of the lake's smaller arthropods, for blood is not essential for their subsistence. Just how the leeches got here in the first place is a puzzling question; none of the other shallow lakes in this guide's area seem to have them. Perhaps one or more were carried up to that environment in relatively recent times by some unfortunate or unsuspecting host. Those interested in aquatic invertebrates will find this lake a well-stocked field laboratory.

To visit Sylvia and Lyons lakes start southwest from the lake along the Bloodsucker Lake Trail. This first descends moderately to a nearby meadow, seasonally rich in wildflowers and mosquitoes, then climbs slightly and briefly southwest to a right angle southeast. On this new tack you pass in 200 yards a shallow, leech-free lake, on your right; then you cross a broad ridge, make a steep ½-mile descent to Lyons Creek, boulder-hop it, and climb east through a meadow to a junction with the Lyons Creek Trail. See Hike 2 for its description up to **Lake Sylvia** and **Lyons Lake**.

Barrett Lake and Red Peak Trails
HIKE 4

Maps
5 and 3

Distances
0.6 mile to Beauty Lake
4.7 miles to Pearl Lake
5.9 miles to Barrett Lake
6.3 miles to Lawrence Lake
6.7 miles to Lake No. 5
6.8 miles to Lake No. 9
6.9 miles to Top Lake
7.3 miles to Lake No. 4
7.6 miles to Lake No. 3

Directions to trailhead

As for Hike 2 take Highway 50 to Wrights Lake Road, which begins 36 miles from Highway 49 in Placerville and 13 miles from Echo Summit. Drive 8.0 miles up this road to a trailhead parking area, on your right, reached just 0.2 mile before the Wrights Lake Information Kiosk. Day users can get wilderness permits here or at trailheads, which are needed for Hikes 4 through 7.

Overnighters must get their permit elsewhere—see Chapter 2's section on wilderness permits. To reach your trailhead, branch left (northwest) immediately past the ranger station and in ¼ mile reach the obvious trailhead with adjacent parking. If you were to continue ⅓ mile farther, you would reach Dark Lake. The limited parking there is for the lake's users, *not* for hikers. You could start from other trailheads in the Wrights Lake area, as well as from the old or new sections of Wrights Lake Campground, and each would give you a different distance to a given point.

Introduction

The Barrett Lake Trail, which is an old jeep road, provides access to an area partly in westernmost Desolation Wilderness that has over a dozen lakes and ponds. This hike describes routes to eight lakes, from popular Barrett Lake to lightly visited Lake No. 9. Just above Barrett Lake is Lawrence Lake, one of our area's more dramatic lakes. Above it is Top Lake, a unique bilobed lake whose water level is two feet higher at its east end than at its west end. And geologically interesting Lake No. 3 provides the start of a cross-country route across the Crystal Range.

Route description

If you go no farther than Barrett Lake, you won't enter the wilderness and won't need a permit. Be aware that every summer OHVs use the jeep roads up to Pearl and Barrett lakes, but only after the roads have become quite drivable. Generally OHVs are allowed from about late July onward, so to avoid motorized recreationists, visit the lakes before then.

Our Rockbound Pass Trail makes a brief climb to a broad, glaciated bedrock ridge and winds north atop it ½ mile to tree-ringed **Beauty Lake**. Large granitic boulders, left by a melting glacier some 14,000 years ago, form miniature islands that add charm to this lake. From here a trail descends south-southeast ⅓ mile to homes by the northwest corner of Wrights Lake. After strolling 70 yards north along Beauty Lake's west shore, we leave the main trail to branch northwest over a nearby gap in a low moraine ridge, and then descend 250 easy yards west to the Barrett Lake (Jeep) Trail.

We start north on the jeep trail, approach the east edge of a pond in 15 yards, and soon descend past the west edge of a larger one, which has grasses and pond lilies. We quickly bottom out to make a fairly level, seasonally muddy traverse ⅓ mile north to a fair campsite, shaded by red firs and lodgepoles, on the east bank of Jones Fork Silver Creek. Where the road crosses the creek, the ford can be up to 15 yards wide, but upstream you can find a boulder hop.

Our road leaves the creek and the forest cover, climbs northwest, and provides us with a view of Rockbound Pass and the adjacent Crystal Range. Soon we reach a wet meadow, rich with wildflowers. Here, in Mortimer Flat, the road splits. For Pearl Lake, take the left fork. This Rupley Jeep Trail climbs ¼ mile through a viewless forest to a broad, equally viewless saddle, then descends north ¼ mile to the northeast edge of a meadow. Where the road turns west to start a climb, the Red Peak Stock Driveway once began a wildly fluctuating 1.5-mile climb to the Barrett Lake Trail. From here onward lies private property of the Rupley Ranch.

The Rupley Jeep Trail next climbs briefly up to a morainal ridge rich in granitic boulders, then descends to a ford of alderchoked Big Silver Creek, which drains the Pearl Lake basin. Beyond the creek we walk about 100 yards west, then follow a spur road northeast ½ mile up glacial sediments to **Pearl Lake**, which lies on Forest Service land. Like almost every lake in the Wrights Lake area, as well as those in adjacent Desolation Wilderness, this

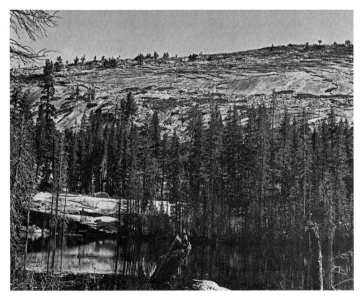

Exfoliation slabs above Pearl Lake

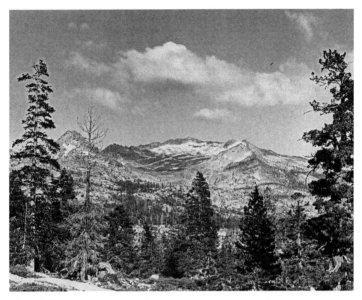

Crystal Range

lake has a low dam, here built to stabilize summer streamflow and to provide a better year-round habitat for fish. Because the lake's water is semistagnant, get fresh water just to the south, at a spring-fed creek.

On the south shore is a fair campsite overlooking the lake's shallow waters, which in the morning reflect the somber, exfoliating slabs above the northeast shore. *Exfoliation* occurs in granitic bedrock because it originally solidified several miles down under pressures on the order of a thousand times more than at the surface. When the overlying material is gone, shells of depressurized granite pop off. Glaciers greatly accelerate the rate of exfoliation, because the Sierra's thick glaciers persisted for thousands of years, adding pressure to the underlying bedrock, and then they rapidly melted away, causing rapid depressurization. Consequently, lots of post-glacial exfoliation occurred, resulting in abundant talus. In contrast, the Sierra's unglaciated granitic lands generally lack talus, for exfoliation occurs so slowly that the resulting rock-fall blocks decompose to gravel before they can accumulate to form a mass of talus.

To reach all the other lakes found along this hike, continue up the Barrett Lake Trail. From Mortimer Flat this jeep trail ascends a little canyon above the flat, curves north up to a low ridge, then fords a wisp of a creek before attaining an open slab from which you'll obtain a panorama of the Crystal Range to the east and southeast. From this vantage point the prominent Wrights Lake and Lyons Creek moraines are very obvious as lateral moraines, whereas close up, their forest cover and their minor irregularities tend to camouflage their shape. Beyond this open slab the jeep trail climbs to a marshy, forested flat, curves east across it, and turns northward up a ridge. This we eventually cross, and then climb steeply up to a saddle and the start of a ridgecrest trail, the Red Peak Stock Driveway. In former years this was used to drive cattle over the Crystal Range and into the heart of Desolation Wilderness. Looking gentle and safe where we see it, this trail becomes, one mile east, a steep, potentially treacherous route. Also, about ½ mile up the driveway a southeast-trending, 1¼-mile-long trail, 16E11, formerly cut across it, linking the Barrett Lake Trail with the Rockbound Pass Trail, passing two shallow lakelets on its way to Willow Flat.

From the ridge the Barrett Lake Trail makes a steep, 0.2-mile descent to a small meadow with a muted creek, this just 30 yards north of the site of former Trail 16E11's northwest end. Across the creek we make a brief, braking descent, then recross its cascading segment. We cross it once more as the jeep road skirts along the east edge of a logged-over meadow being invaded by lodgepoles. Just past the turn of the century this plot was sold by the Barrett family to the University of California at Davis, which set up an experimental station here and tried to improve the local herds through selective breeding. From this site we climb, steeply in places, to a broad saddle, on which our jeep road diminishes to a trail. After a short, sunny, gravelly descent we reach the swift Barrett Lake outlet creek, a boulder hop. Now we follow a gully that in places becomes a shallow chute, and in ¼ mile the jeep trail ends at an enormous, flat campsite, under shady red firs, occupying most of the west shore of **Barrett Lake**. This site would hold a large Boy Scout troop with room to spare, and its coves and diving rocks, together with its shallow rock-slab pools below its low dam, would keep all the kids active and content.

Beyond Barrett Lake we take the Red Peak Trail, which doesn't go to the peak. This begins as a pack trail, first climbing steeply 0.1 mile to the wilderness boundary, then steeply up another 0.1 mile to a trail junction by the cascading Lawrence Lake outlet creek. Now with law-abiding OHVers staying behind at Barrett Lake, we branch right for an easy creekside climb to a fair campsite near the northwest end of the waist-high dam across **Lawrence Lake**. Cross the dam and take a footpath past a small rock island to Top Lake's outlet creek, which announces itself 150 yards before

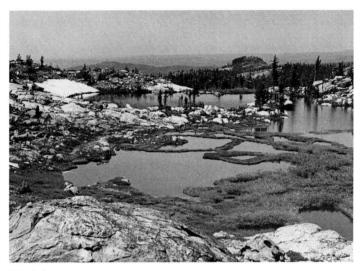

Top Lake

entering the beautiful, symmetrical lake by cascading 50 feet down a glistening rock slab. To the east is the higher but less spectacular cascade of the outlet creek of **Lake No. 9**. A ½ mile walk up along either creek will get you to less used campsites at these two lakes.

A side trip to **Top Lake** is particularly rewarding. Perched at the lip of a cirque, it seems to sit on top of the world, and the backpacker who sets up camp here enjoys panoramic sunsets that are hard to match anywhere. The lake has a peninsula that almost divides it in two. The most amazing aspect of the lake, however, is its naturally terraced east end, where water is ponded up as much as 2 feet higher than at the west end. Thick clumps of grass and heather are progressively invading the lake, building dikes and trapping sediments. More vegetation grows upon them and ponds up the water level.

For more lake hunting, return to the Red Peak Trail junction. If you contour ¼ mile southwest from it, you reach a bench holding shallow Lost Lake, probably the least visited of the Red Peak lakes. Keeping to the trail, climb steeply north 0.2 mile to a forested ridge, then make a short descent to a meadow in which you pass three seasonal ponds, all on your right. Flowing from the last of these, as well as from a soggy meadow, is a small creek we must cross before it enters **Lake No. 5**. This lake is a haunt of spotted sandpipers, who build nests in the dense grass along the water's edge. If you want to camp at this serene lake, do so on the west shore, a dry, rocky moraine from which you obtain tree-framed views down the glaciated slopes to the west.

Beyond the lake we climb to a saddle, where our trail turns abruptly right. The ducked path straight ahead leads 0.2 mile northwest down to unappealing, semistagnant **Lake No. 4.** Our trail climbs north-northeast up an open, bedrock slope to a narrow ridge. If not well marked, this stretch can be missed. The correct route goes through a shallow gap in the narrow ridge and continues 50 yards beyond it to a junction. From here the Red Peak Trail drops northwest 1½ miles—very steeply at times—to the western edge of Map 3, crossing Lake No. 3's outlet creek near this point. It then continues another 1½ miles down to the western boundary of Desolation Wilderness and heads west about 3 miles to the Van Vieck trailhead. Taking this route in would be a slightly shorter route to Lake Nos. 3 and 4, but longer to all others.

With Lake No. 3 as the last goal along Hike 4, we leave the Red Peak Trail just beyond the narrow ridge and hike northeast through a swampy meadow, head between a rock pile on the left and the main rock slope on the right, and curve northward up to another wet, spongy meadow through which flows the tiny outlet creek from Lake No. 3. Small though it is, this creek can support good-size trout. Across the creek we head northwest toward the base of a moraine at a point 30 yards west of the creek's cas-

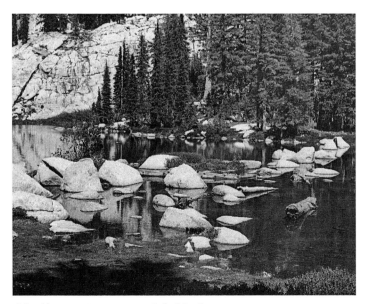

A bouldery moraine cuts across Lake No. 3

cade. Now it's just a short climb up to **Lake No. 3**, whose relative isolation from Wrights Lake rewards you with relatively pristine lakeside campsites beneath a cover of mountain hemlock and lodgepole and western white pines. Those wishing to spend a few days here might make a relatively easy cross-country day hike northeast to the saddle between Red Peak and Silver Peak, and then descend to the Leland Lakes.

Hikers content to relax at lovely Lake No. 3 might take note of the arc of boulders near its outlet, which make up a recessional moraine—one formed behind a glacier's terminal moraine. Lake No. 3 stands out from others in that it has a clear recessional moraine behind the more amorphous one found at the lake's outlet. Many Sierra lakes appear to be dammed by such recessional moraines, but actually it is the bedrock beneath the moraine that is damming them. When you return to Wrights Lake, walk to its picnic area, north along the shore of this surprisingly shallow large lake, and see how many recessional moraines you can identify.

Twin Lakes and Grouse Lake Trails

HIKE 5

Maps

5

Distances

2.1 miles to Grouse Lake

2.6 miles to Hemlock Lake

2.7 miles to Lower Twin Lake

3.0 miles to Smith Lake

3.1 miles to Upper Twin and Boomerang lakes

3.3 miles to Island Lake

Directions to trailhead

See directions for Hike 4. To reach the trailhead, branch right just past the Wrights Lake Information Kiosk, passing the entrance to the new Wrights Lake Campground, then past homes to a fairly large trailhead parking area, on your right. The actual trailhead is just down the road, at its turnaround.

Introduction

Because these attractive lakes lie so close to Wrights Lake, they receive heavy use. Therefore, to minimize your impact at these lakes, please make day hikes to them rather than camp overnight at them, for they aren't that hard to hike to. Although the lakes are close together, each is unique, having its own special attributes. From Smith Lake, the highest, you obtain one of the best trail views of the Wrights Lake and Crystal Basin recreation areas.

Route description

Three trails leave from the road's end by the east arm of Wrights Lake. One begins west along the arm and eventually bifurcates, one branch going to an amphitheater and to the southeastern Wrights Lake Campground, the other going to the lake's dam. Another trail crosses a prominent bridge over the lake's inlet creek. From the bridge's far side, one branch strikes west along the lake's north shore, while another goes first northwest then north to a road from which the old Rockbound Pass Trail still begins an ascent. The third branch—yours—meanders northeastward, keeping just within forest cover to avoid a swampy meadow just to the west. After 0.4 mile of easy walking, you reach a trail. This trail starts northwest, then heads west over to the old Rockbound Pass Trail.

From the junction you take the Twin Lakes Trail for a climb quite steadily northeast, often within hearing distance of Grouse Lake's outlet creek. After a mile of climbing, you reach another junction, from which the Grouse Lake Trail (formerly the Hemlock Lakes Trail) continues east up to Grouse, Hemlock, and Smith lakes, described later in this hike.

Keeping on the Twin Lakes Trail, you branch left (north) and immediately cross Grouse Lake's outlet creek. Next, you climb north up quite open glacier-polished slabs, then bend northeast for a curving ascent moderately up additional slabs. Soon the trail heads north over a minor ridge, then traverses northeast before climbing east along Twin Lakes' outlet creek. From a boggy area crossed on large-block stepping stones, you make a short climb northeast to **Lower Twin Lake**, whose outlet creek the trail crosses about 40 yards below a waist-high dam. You may find it more convenient to cross immediately below the dam. Before you cross, however, you might want to stop at the lake's south shore and rest awhile or swim and dive from rocks along this fairly deep shore. Anglers will find the lake stocked with trout. Rainbow trout were first introduced in 1904 by Joe Minghetti, a local hand, who eventually stocked most of the lakes in the Wrights Lake Recreation Area.

From the dam the trail parallels the lake's west shore to a gully at its northwest corner, from where you could climb west to a low nearby ridge for views and then descend to compact Umpa Lake. But with Boomerang Lake in mind, stick to the Twin Lakes Trail, which is now faint and rocky. It climbs northeast from the gully, passes through a 10-foot-deep notch, then reaches **Boomerang Lake**, on whose north shore of the southeast arm one can dive from 12-foot ledges into the lake's often cold, deep water. By descending southeast cross-country, you can quickly reach the north shore of **Upper Twin Lake**, which is a mere 2 feet higher than its sibling. Glacier-polished, gently sloping slabs separate the twins, and in this vicinity lie fair campsites.

After passing between Boomerang Lake and its northeastern satellite, the Twin Lakes Trail climbs above the northern end

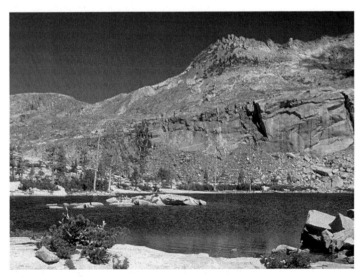

Lower Twin Lake

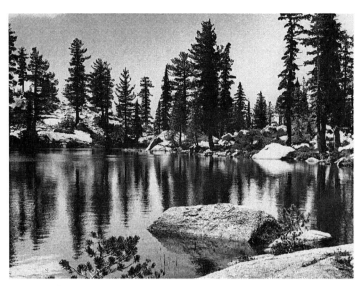

Grouse Lake

of a small, linear lake, fed by a seasonal snowfield and by two longer-lasting, narrow cascades from Island Lake. In a brief climb you reach **Island Lake**, a fairly large, rock-island lake whose shores are nearly devoid of trees. Although tall, dark-gray diorite-gabbro cirque walls lend a stark beauty to this alpine lake, it is not as popular as the Twin Lakes, with their border of sparse trees. At Island Lake you may find more gulls or ducks than backpackers. From this lake accomplished mountaineers can strike northwest over a saddle and descend to Tyler and Gertrude lakes (Hike 6), or strike southeast for a more arduous ascent of Mt. Price, which at 9975 feet is only 8 feet less than the wilderness' highest, Pyramid Peak.

To reach Grouse, Hemlock, and Smith lakes, take the Grouse Lake Trail. In about 100 yards it enters Desolation Wilderness, following a ducked route up granitic slabs into an open forest and to a gravelly flat. The trail turns southeast and then starts to climb more gradually, but soon it becomes steep, and after a brief traverse to cross a creek, it continues steeply but briefly up to a moraine at the outlet of **Grouse Lake**. This lake, fringed with rocks, meadow, red mountain heather and Labrador tea, is a very pleasant lake to linger at or swim in—after early August, when the mosquitoes have greatly abated. Nearby campsites, on sloping ground above its northeast shore, should be avoided; better sites exist above the far shore, and you can reach them by a use trail that circles the lake. Leaky, fish-free Secret Lake, reached by a short cross-county hike south from Grouse Lake, is a disappointment.

A steep climb north up a low ridge with glacial deposits plus a longer ascent northeast up a rocky slope bring us to tiny **Hemlock Lake,** named for the mountain hemlocks that border its south shore. Its small size is compensated for by a dramatic exfoliating cliff above its north shore.

Hiking southeast, we make a final ducked climb, the last bit steep and blocky, and reach **Smith Lake,** which at 8700 feet is almost at treeline. Its steep, confining slopes, most having snowfields that last well into the summer, also retard tree growth. Nevertheless, a small stand of lodgepole and western white pines thrives above the lake's northwest shore. From a rocky spot near the lake's outlet we can view the Wrights Lake and Crystal Basin recreation areas and identify Wrights Lake and Dark Lake below us and Union Valley Reservoir in the distance. This is the only lake from which you can get such expansive views of these two areas. No adequate campsite exists at the lake.

Tyler Lake Trail

HIKE 6

Maps
5 and 3

Distances
3.8 miles to Gertrude Lake
3.9 miles to Tyler Lake

Directions to trailhead
Same directions as for Hike 5.

Introduction

Two photogenic subalpine lakes climax this moderate hike. Despite their somewhat easy accessibility, they remain relatively unvisited, perhaps because hikers prefer the closer lakes of Hike 5 or the "backcountry" ones beyond Rockbound Pass. If you are in good shape, lower your environmental impact by making this route a day hike.

Route description

This hike begins from the Twin Lakes trailhead by the east arm of Wrights Lake. Alternatively, you could use the Rockbound trailhead (Hike 4), though doing so would increase your hike by about ½ mile. Our trail begins by crossing a prominent bridge over the lake's inlet creek. From the bridge's far side, a use trail heads west to north-shore homes, while our trail heads first northwest, then north, staying within forest cover to avoid a seasonally swampy meadow. Here Ed Wright grazed his dairy cattle from 1850 to 1900, and cattle still graze once it dries out. After 0.4 mile our trail, now widened to a road, meets a trail eastbound for the Twin Lakes (Hike 5). In about 15 yards our road starts a curve west and meets a spur road. If you continued west about 90 yards, you would reach a trail that climbs west to Beauty Lake.

We take the spur road north, the start of the old Rockbound Pass Trail, and over ⅓ mile it quickly narrows to a trail and then reaches a junction with a trail that climbs southwest to Beauty Lake. Keeping north we can enjoy the nearly level tread for ¼ mile, then make a generally moderate climb ⅓ mile to a ridge junction with the new Rockbound Pass Trail. United, our trail climbs northeast on old tread, first shortly up the ridge, then below and north of it to reach, in about ½ mile, a junction in a small, shady flat. From here we follow the Tyler Lake Trail to its end at, surprisingly, Gertrude Lake.

Climbing east above the flat, we quickly enter Desolation Wilderness as we follow this ducked trail up slabs and a gully to a viewpoint, from where we can trace the outlet streams of Umpa and Twin Lakes flowing—sometimes cascading—over open, glaciated slabs on their way down to Wrights Lake. Our trail drops briefly to a flat, then climbs north steeply up a brush-lined gully to a forested, shallow saddle on a ridge. Beyond it the trail parallels an ephemeral creeklet and then climbs steeply north above it, becoming faint before reaching another ridge. From a shallow saddle, it enters a hemlock forest, with an ankle-deep pond, then makes a fluctuating traverse northeast. Blazes and ducks guide our route across snow-fed creeklets, and then we make a steep, bouldery ascent to a short spur trail, which descends a willow-choked gully 125 yards to Tyler's grave. A local ranch hand, he froze to death in a November 1882 snowstorm while trying to round up cattle. Along a 0.2-mile ascent bisected by Tyler Lake's creek, our trail becomes faint before reaching **Gertrude Lake**. Short on campsites but long on scenery, this shallow lake has a photogenic balance of shoreline slabs and spaced conifers.

To reach our trail's namesake, backtrack to its creek and parallel it up open slabs to **Tyler Lake**. Only a few scattered pines and hemlocks provide shade at this slab-happy lake, which lies in an alpine setting. Exposed but legal campsites lie above its rocky east shore.

Rockbound Pass Trail

HIKE 7

Maps

5 and 3

Distances

0.6 mile to Beauty Lake

4.6 miles to Maud Lake

5.9 miles to Rockbound Pass

6.2 miles to Lake Doris

7.3 miles to Lake Lois

8.6 miles to Lake Schmidell

9.8 miles to lower Leland Lake

10.6 miles to McConnell Lake

10.8 miles to Camper Flat

11.8 miles to Horseshoe Lake

12.0 miles to 4-Q Lakes (via Camper Flat)

12.3 miles to Lake Zitella

13.5 miles to Highland Lake

13.9 miles to 4-Q Lakes (via McConnell Lake)

Directions to trailhead

See directions for Hike 4.

Introduction

Some visitors will only want to make a 9.2-mile day hike to Maud Lake and back. Unfortunately, when too many people linger at Maud Lake, it is likely to metamorphose to "Mud Lake." It's probably the most popular trailside lake reached from Wrights Lake trailheads. If you go beyond Rockbound Pass, you'll probably want to make your trek an overnighter. Weekend backpackers usually venture only as far as Lake Lois or Schmidell. Those fortunate enough to have the time to visit every lake along this hike will log 29.6 miles, and should allow at least four days to properly savor the route's many delights.

Route description

As on Hike 4, we take the Rockbound Pass Trail briefly up to a broad, glaciated bedrock ridge and wind north atop it ½ mile to tree-ringed **Beauty Lake**. We head 70 yards north along its west shore, to where a trail, Hike 4, branches northwest over a minor gap. Then we curve eastward about 250 yards, exit north through another gap and, just east and up from it, meet a trail fork. Right, a trail descends eastward to the Twin Lakes Trail (Hike 5). We go left to wind 300 yards northeast up to another trail fork in a shallow, forested ridge saddle, from which a lightly used trail descends northeast to the old Rockbound Pass Trail. Rather than drop, only to climb again, we take the new trail, which weaves along both sides of an irregular ridge, providing views both east and west. In about 0.9 mile we rejoin the old trail, and on an old tread climb northeast, first shortly up the ridge, then below and north of it to reach, in about ½ mile, a junction in a small, shady flat. From here the Tyler Lake Trail (Hike 6) climbs, surprisingly, to Gertrude Lake.

Our Rockbound Pass Trail branches left, crosses several snowmelt creeklets, soon enters Desolation Wilderness, then climbs moderately-to-steeply ½ mile north through a thinning forest to a seasonal pond atop a saddle. Now the trail makes an equally long and steep descent across brushy slabs to a boulder crossing

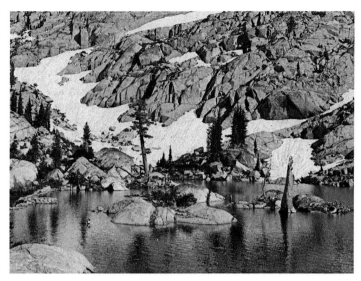

Highland Lake

of Jones Fork Silver Creek 1¼ miles below Maud Lake. Beyond the crossing the rock-lined trail ascends largely barren, low-angle, glacially polished and striated slabs upon which rest numerous erratic boulders left by a retreating glacier. Along the massive slabs' sparse fractures grow junipers, lodgepoles, and other plants that can get a roothold.

We cross a low, minor ridge, parallel it north, and enter the thicket of Willow Flat, which besides willows has bracken ferns, corn lilies, and aspens. A short, bouldery, creekside ascent leads to a shady flat, where we cross a seasonal creek just below its rush down a polished ramp. We make a shady ascent 200 yards to within several yards of the forest's abrupt north edge, from where Trail 16E11 once traversed westward over to two shallow, unappealing lakelets before intersecting the Red Peak Stock Driveway and ending at the Barrett Lake (Jeep) Trail (Hike 4).

Climbing toward Maud Lake, our trail leaves forest shade behind as it switchbacks up a barren slope, traverses northeast above Silver Creek's inner gorge, and then makes a short descent to a pond. Immediately above it lies **Maud Lake**. Campsites abound, many illegal, around this popular lake. Overuse by both hikers and packers has impacted the lake, and its water today is semiclear and definitely should be treated before drinking. Swimmers who venture out in its relatively warm, shallow water can attest to the muddy character of the lake's bottom, which may have prompted someone to remove the *a* in a former *Maud Lake* sign (in the 1990s the spelling changed from Maud to Maude but USFS maps, and the author's, still show it as Maud).

Ahead lies a 900-foot elevation gain to Rockbound Pass. This is not a major gain by High Sierra standards, but it is for Desolation Wilderness. For some the ascent is intimidating because you almost always see the stark pass looming up before you, and because its dwarf trees make it look higher and farther away than it is. Our trail to the pass was built around 1918, after an early heavy October storm of the previous year almost decimated a herd of cattle then grazing in and above Rockbound Valley. Joe Minghetti, a hired hand on the Blakely Ranch but formerly a Swiss stone mason, was commissioned by the Forest Service to build the trail so that there would be an escape route for the cattle when they had to be quickly evacuated. The trail was not to exceed 15° in grade, but as the hiker soon finds out, in places it does.

The climb from Maud Lake starts out through a sloping meadow, which is boggy for most of the summer, and then goes steeply up slopes abundant with huckleberry oak, western service-berry, and wildflowers. The trail's switchbacks—short and steep—are characteristic of old, pre-recreation standards, when trails were made as steep as the stock would bear. After the last set of switchbacks we reach a small flat with several large junipers growing on and near it. From this welcome rest spot you can appreciate the progress you've made, and can enjoy views of the nearby head of your canyon, and of Maud Lake in the middle distance, forested lands beyond.

Also in sight are three granitic plutons, originally formed several miles below the earth's surface. Long ago each of three light-density molten masses worked its way up through existing rock until it finally cooled to form a solid mass, a pluton. On the wall opposite you, from north to south, the three plutons are orange, dark gray, and light gray, and their respective compositions are granite, diorite-gabbro, and probably granodiorite.

Beyond the junipers you almost stroll up to sometimes windy **Rockbound Pass**, with its weather-beaten, dwarfed mountain hemlocks and lodgepole and whitebark pines. Typically snow-bound through late July, the trail from this pass switchbacks northeast down toward Lake Doris, passing both red mountain heather and white heather. Note that not only are their flowers different colors, they are differently shaped, and the former has needle-like leaves while the latter has scale-like ones. Both grow in prime-mosquito areas—something to think about should you ever camp near them. Among hemlocks growing above the lake's north shore is a fair campsite. After briefly touching the east shore of shallow **Lake Doris**—the turf here sometimes painted yellow with buttercups and marsh marigolds—the trail climbs a few feet, then makes a brief descent to a junction. From here the Rockbound Pass Trail descends 1½ miles east down to Rockbound Valley (see end of Hike 10).

Our trail, the Blakely Trail, descends northwest to immediately cross Lake Doris' outlet creek, then makes a scenic traverse north, offering us panoramas to the east. It passes just above one lakelet and then skirts two ponds on a low, broad saddle, and quickly reaches an east finger of **Lake Lois**. This lake rests in a basin mostly of dark diorite-gabbro bedrock, although its southern part and the lower cliffs above it are varying hues of marine sandstone that was metamorphosed through repeated, compressive forces acting on the area.

Popular Lake Lois and its neighbor one mile to the northwest, Lake Schmidell, both bear the brunt of weekend backpackers. At each you'll find many sites that are within 100 feet of the shore and very few that are more than 100 feet away. Imaginative backpackers can find additional, isolated sites on small, level benches east and north of Lake Lois. This lake's southeast corner, although often only 50°F in mid-August, attracts some who like to do brisk high diving—up to 20+ feet—into its very deep water. Those who just like to swim will find its isolated east finger 10° warmer. The lake is stocked, but given its high usage, don't count on a trout meal.

Paralleling the east finger, the rocky trail winds over to the outlet creek, crosses its low dam, heads briefly west along the north shore, and then climbs north ⅓ mile to a ridge, where it meets the Red Peak Stock Driveway. This old stock trail climbs 1¼ miles to a high, but shallow, gap on the Crystal Range crest. It then descends about 2 miles—dangerously steep in one 400-foot drop— to the Barrett Lake (Jeep) Trail (Hike 4). The stock driveway is an occasionally scenic route back to Wrights Lake that is best left to competent hikers who want to take "the route less traveled by."

From the stock-driveway junction we make a fairly steep descent northwest through an open forest, almost touching a small creek before reaching a junction not far from **Lake Schmidell**. To reach its campsites you could hike northeast 200 yards down a trail to a pond, then 250 yards northwest up to the lake's dammed outlet creek. An easier way to reach its campsites, which are perched on a mountain-hemlock-and-lodgepole-shaded bench above the southeast shore, is to walk due north 100 yards from the junction.

This junction is the start of a 9.6-mile loop that, clockwise, visits lower Leland Lake, McConnell Lake, Horseshoe Lake and its Highland Lake Trail junction, 4-Q Lakes, Camper Flat, and Lake Schmidell. The first part of this loop, along the McConnell Lake Trail, reaches the Highland Lake Trail junction in only 3½ miles. This part is the shorter, and the more scenic and popular way to the junction, and so will be described first.

The McConnell Lake Trail leaves the junction above Lake Schmidell and first traverses southwest to a cascading creek. You boulder-hop it, then make a scenic though taxing ascent to a shallow saddle on the granodiorite ridge above Lake Schmidell's talus slopes. The Leland Lakes quickly come into view as we make an equally steep descent north toward the upper lake. Avoiding this lake's grassy east shore, our trail swings northeast a bit, dips through a boggy meadow, and then descends to the southeast corner of **lower Leland Lake**. Since its lakeshore campsites are off limits, you might look for a site on land between the two Leland Lakes. Camping here is definitely inferior to that at Lakes Schmidell and Lois.

Leaving the lower lake, we descend alongside its cheerful outlet creek, cross it in a forested flat, and continue briefly northwest to the forest's edge. Watching for ducks—both the rock kind and in late season the live ones—we follow a path that arcs around the west shore of a marshy pond, **McConnell Lake**. Most campers will avoid it, so the few that linger in the environs are likely to have solitude. Leaving its soggy meadow of grass and heather behind, we reach a low ridge, head through a few yards of brush, and then descend an open slope northwest to the base of an imposing granodiorite wall, which would provide challenging ascents to any climber willing to haul in ropes and gear.

A prominent low-angle waterfall glides down the middle of this wall, and just after crossing its creek on level ground, one can encounter route-finding problems. If you do, look for ducks that mark the route up and down a low slab. Then just beyond it, where the trail climbs over another low slab to a gully with a trickling creek, contour east 100 yards, descend slightly to another short traverse, this one northeast, then top a low, rocky ridge. Several short switchbacks lead down to an alluvial flat on which lies shallow **Horseshoe Lake**, speckled with rock islands. Although you may not find a legal campsite along the lake, you can find many legal ones on the small flats of the low ridge south-

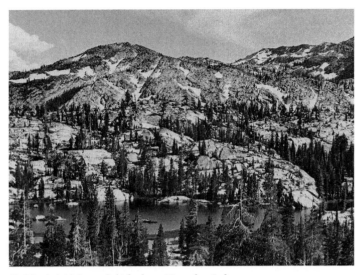

Red Peak (right) stands high above Horseshoe Lake

east of the lake. Being quite open, the ridge provides campers with very scenic, panoramic views.

Just above the northeast corner of Horseshoe Lake is a junction with the Highland Lake Trail. Before describing it, this guidebook now will describe the long, counterclockwise way to this junction.

This generally viewless route first drops 200 yards to the pond below Lake Schmidell's outlet creek, staying on the Blakely Trail as it makes an eastward, heather-lined descent—muddy and mosquito-ridden usually through mid-August—to a crossing of the outlet creek. Immediately beyond this it reaches a lateral, the Schmidell Trail, for those traveling to upper Rockbound Valley, Mosquito Pass, and Lake Aloha. Beyond this junction you make an equally long, but drier, descent to a second crossing, then in ⅓ mile reach a junction on a bench above the Rubicon River. One hundred yards south of this junction a trail fords the Rubicon and then climbs east to Middle Velma Lake and over to Lake Tahoe's Highway 89 (Hikes 19, 20, and 23).

Start north along the Rubicon and in 70 yards reach a spur trail west to a cold, rusty, seeping mineral spring. After a few minutes winding walk north, you reach broad, level **Camper Flat**, where beside a good, if brisk, Rubicon swimming hole is a campsite. Bearing westward through a lush meadow, you reach your last crossing of Lake Schmidell's outlet creek. If necessary, look for a log to cross it and then reach in 70 yards, near open slabs lining the Rubicon, the McConnell Lake Trail. This west-climbing trail skirts several stagnant ponds before reaching the first small lake of the relatively warm **4-Q Lakes,** this one about 40 yards northwest of the trail (an orphaned 4-Q Lake lies south of the trail, just on the other side of a short, low, broad ridge.) Just ¼ mile beyond it is the second 4-Q lake, across which you must "walk on water." Two peninsulas almost cut the lake in half, and you cross the shallow, 40-foot strait via rocks and/or logs.

Beyond the lake crossing the trail curves over to the west shore of this lake, touches upon the north shore of adjacent lake number three, and then makes a brief climb to a stagnant, bush-fringed pond, where you often do have to walk on the water to follow the trail. Most hikers keep their feet dry by going around and above the pond's edge and then rejoining the trail, which climbs a few paces before descending southwest to the fourth lake, subjectively the best. In the fairly open forest in the 4-Q Lakes area, there are plenty of small bedrock benches ideal for an isolated camp.

From the north end of the fourth lake the ducked route goes along the lake's outlet-creek gully, first descending moderately northwest through red-fir stands, then it eases its grade and descends north through alternating lodgepole-pine stands and huckleberry-oak scrub. Nearing the end of this 1.4-mile descent,

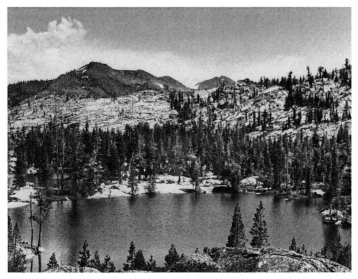

Dicks Peak (center) pokes above the third 4-Q Lake

we find ourselves often walking along glaciated granodiorite slabs. Watch carefully for ducks. Our trail crosses the creek just 20 yards above a narrow chute you can jump across. In this vicinity you can find rocky campsites whose hardness is more than compensated for by their isolation and by the nearby views north down the Rubicon River's canyon, Rockbound Valley.

Now climbing west, it is important to follow the ducks if you want to minimize your effort. The often faint trail climbs steeply up a slope, staying about 100-200 yards north of Horseshoe Lake's outlet creek. The route reaches a ridge above that lake, and then you follow ducks for about 50 yards west down to the Highland Lake Trail junction, mentioned earlier.

To visit Lake Zitella and Highland Lake, take this trail, which climbs steeply up a gully. Above it you diagonal left up more-open slabs, from which you have a backward glance at photogenic Horseshoe Lake and its dramatic backdrop, the spine of the Crystal Range. Notice how the trees on the granitic slopes beyond the lake are concentrated along *master joints*, which are major fracture lines in this otherwise very resistant rock. Our 200-foot ascent tops out at a saddle, from which the trail ahead to alluring Lake Zitella descends ¼ mile to this shallow lake's outlet creek. Just before crossing it, look northeast across Rockbound Valley. If the master joints above Horseshoe Lake weren't obvious, hopefully the ones on the opposite canyon wall are unmistakably clear.

Relatively shallow, slightly cloudy **Lake Zitella** is one of the warmest cirque lakes in the wilderness, its temperature rising into the low 70s. It is an excellent swimming hole, with plenty of shoreline slabs and rock islands to bask on. In the shallow water, yellow-legged frogs, unlike trout, are sometimes abundant. Several campsites exist, these above the west half of the lake. Above the lake is a low-angle cliff that provides easy routes for rock climbers.

Those seeking isolation can now begin an arduous route to Highland Lake. The northwest-bound trail climbing from Lake Zitella's north shore is simple enough, but from the saddle above it, the trail makes an extremely steep descent—almost an uncontrolled slide at times—down a gully. Despite its steepness, it is not very exposed and not very dangerous. This steep route exists because a cliff prevents a traverse west. At the base of the cliff the route turns west and begins to climb. At this point one views an obvious, open, cross-country route, spread out below, descending to either Rockbound Lake or Rubicon Reservoir (Hike 1).

Hiking toward Highland Lake, watch for ducks that mark the open rock-slab ascent to a crossing of Highland Lake creek at the lip of a cirque, then traverse 150 yards southwest to the northeast shore of a rockbound lakelet. From it the trail makes a winding, ducked ascent in the same direction up to a ridge that is just north of a tiny, photogenic lakelet, whose waters are aerated by several cascades splashing into it. After a momentary descent, we make a short, steep ascent to a shelf, which we follow briefly south to icy, trout-stocked **Highland Lake**. Being rockbound, it has only small campsites that are fair at best. Also being the wilderness' most remote lake by trail, it has the *potential* for solitude.

Horsetail Falls Trail

HIKE 8

Maps   *Distances*

6   1.4 miles to base of lower Horsetail Fall

          1.9 miles to Avalanche Lake

          2.1 miles to Pitt Lake

          2.5 miles to Ropi Lake

          3.6 miles to Lake of the Woods

          5.0 miles to Lake Aloha, southeast corner

Directions to trailhead

From the Highway 49 junction in Placerville, drive 5 miles east up Highway 50 to the Eldorado National Forest Information Center, get your wilderness permit there, then continue 35 miles up the highway to the settlement of Strawberry. Finally, drive an additional 1.6 miles to the signed, paved Pyramid Creek trailhead, an obvious trailhead parking area at the site of former Twin Bridges. The parking area entrance is about 200 yards west of and before the highway's bridge over Pyramid Creek. (Westbound drivers: this parking area is 6.8 miles west from Echo Summit.) There are more than 40 parking spaces, and on summer weekends, all may be taken, attesting to the trail's popularity. Be aware that there is a daily parking fee, which was $3 in 2002, but could increase.

Introduction

Pyramid Creek is an understandably popular trailhead, for the trail from it provides the quickest route to the Desolation Valley lakes. An official trail exists only to the wilderness' boundary, and beyond that the route essentially is cross country. This is the only dangerous route described in this book, and it would not be described at all were it not an official way into the wilderness. Supposedly a number of hikers have fallen to their deaths trying to reach Desolation Valley.

Route description

If you need a guidebook to stay on route, you shouldn't be on this sketchy trail. Consequently, the directions for it are intentionally very brief. Also, if you haven't hiked it, don't do so alone—you might have to be rescued.

From an obvious trailhead, the trail winds about 400 yards east to the west side of Pyramid Creek, joining it about 0.1 mile north of the Highway 50 bridge. You quickly leave the creek near its bend east, then rejoin it ½ mile later and follow it 250 yards northwest through open forest to another bend, then 160 yards north to the wilderness boundary, in a shady fir grove. About ½ mile past the boundary your first real route-finding problems begin, and if you can't find the trail, turn back; it gets worse ahead. After about 200 yards of climbing up an increasingly steep tread, you reach a vantage point from which you can look down-canyon and identify the canyon's huge east-wall lateral moraine. You can also study nearby **lower Horsetail Fall**, often roaring as it plunges 100 feet into a splashing pool. This vantage point is on ice- and water-polished, gravel-covered, sloping bedrock. In other words, it's very slippery. One could easily slip and plunge on a one-way trip into the lower fall's rocky gorge.

The trail, if you can call it that, veers away from the lower fall and starts west steeply up open slabs. In several places you'll probably have to use your hands as well as your feet. And you'll have to use good judgment in route finding. High above the lower fall the route bends north and diagonals up a talus slope before cutting 80 yards east to a small flat just above the brink of upper Horsetail Fall. The view from the flat *almost* justifies this arduous

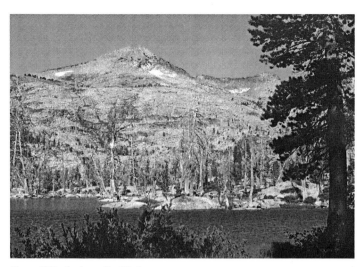

Pyramid Peak above Ropi Lake

ascent, and from it you can now identify the canyon's west-wall moraine, which isn't nearly so spectacular as its multistage east-wall counterpart. It's hard to believe that a glacier descending Pyramid Creek filled the canyon at least to the crest of these 900-foot-high moraines.

With danger behind you, drop briefly north from the small flat, then parallel Pyramid Creek 200 yards up to small but scenic **Avalanche Lake.** Your route to Ropi Lake is now essentially cross-country. About ¼ mile beyond Avalanche Lake you approach relatively unappealing **Pitt Lake,** and near its northern end you must make a decision. To get to Lake of the Woods, you'll have to cross Pyramid Creek, and this is best done before you reach Ropi Lake—if you want to keep your feet dry. Therefore, start looking for suitable boulders and/or logs on which you can cross the creek.

The principal cross-country route stays along the creek's west bank as it climbs ⅓ mile to the outlet of **Ropi Lake.** From here, one can head west to nearby Toem Lake or, above it, to Gefo Lake. For solitude seekers, isolated lakelets and ponds lie on naked granite to the south of these. A fast way to Lake Aloha is to climb north from Toem or Gefo, passing Pyramid and Waca lakes. You can also start from Ropi Lake's northeast shore and ascend Pyramid Creek, passing a chain of lakes up to Lake Aloha's principal dam.

From the east arm of snag-infested Ropi Lake, an official trail starts a climb to Lake of the Woods. This trail ascends east-northeast ⅓ mile up a joint-controlled gully, crosses a tiny, seasonally boggy flat, then continues on an easier grade ¼ mile east to Lake of the Woods outlet creek. This it follows 200 yards upstream to a crossing that can be hard to find for those *descending* this trail. From the crossing you head east immediately past the south edge of a small, stagnant pond, then immediately turn north to begin a ¼-mile climb to a low ridge damming extremely popular **Lake of the Woods**. This lake's shores abound with campsites, the better, more private ones being found along its west shore. If you camp here, be sure you do so *at least* 100 feet from the shore—200 feet is better.

At the lake's northwest corner, which is nearly a mile by trail from its outlet, take a trail that starts a climb northwest, reaching a popular trail to Lake Aloha in less than ½ mile. Just 60 yards down it you reach a junction above a southeast arm of shallow, sprawling **Lake Aloha**. From here a popular *de facto* trail branches left and embarks on a ¾-mile course over to the lake's 20-foot-high dam. Relatively warm in August and dotted with islands, the part of the lake near the dam is a justifiably popular swimming area. On barren granitic benches to the south of the lake you can make a camp.

Ralston Peak Trail
HIKE 9

Maps
6

Distance
4.0 miles to Ralston Peak

Directions to trailhead

From the Pyramid Creek Trailhead, mentioned in the previous hike's trailhead description, drive 1¼ miles up Highway 50 to Camp Sacramento, on your right, and Sayles Flat, on your left.

(Westbound drivers, this spot is 5¾ miles west from Echo Summit.) Park on the flat if there is no room at the trailhead. To reach it, head 200 yards up an old, paved road to a chapel. Immediately beyond it the road curves sharply right, and the trail begins from it.

Introduction

You'll command excellent views, both nearby and far-reaching, from the summit of Ralston Peak. From it you can study the different characteristics of Desolation Wilderness, the river canyons to the west, the Carson Range to the northeast, and the Freel Peak area to the east.

You can reach Ralston's summit by the overly steep Ralston Peak Trail or by the moderately graded Pacific Crest Trail (Hike 10) from Echo Lake. The "PCT" route is about 3 miles longer, but its trailhead is 1000 feet higher, which means you have a lot less effort. Furthermore, you can cut 2½ miles off the PCT route by taking the Echo Lakes water taxi, thereby making it the shorter and the easier of the two routes. The Ralston Peak Trail may appeal only to hikers wanting a physical challenge.

Route description

From the road's sharp curve your trail begins by switch-backing up through a white-fir forest that shades the slopes of a giant lateral moraine. The trail almost tops the level crest of the moraine but chooses instead to parallel it for about 200 yards before actually reaching it. From this spot you can gaze northwest at pointed Pyramid Peak, which stands high above 900-foot-deep, glaciated Pyramid Creek canyon below you. To the southwest lies the nearly vertical west face of Lovers Leap (Hike 25), a popular climbing area. Along the stretch of trail just before and after this viewpoint you may see one or more faint trails climbing up to yours. These start from a church camp in Pinecrest.

Now you face a steep-to-very-steep 1350-foot open climb up weathered granitic rock that is largely covered with huckleberry oak, manzanita, and some chinquapin. A 60-yard-long spur trail marks the 500-foot point. Continued steep climbing up short switchbacks for an elevation gain of 450 feet brings us to an eastward traverse, along which we pass a trickling spring. A few more short, steep switchbacks are negotiated, and then the gradient eases as we climb to a prominent spur ridge, covered with an open stand of red firs and western white pines. From it a brief initial descent speeds us on our way along a ⅓-mile traverse northwest across a meadowy slope.

Just after our traverse turns into a moderate climb, we encounter two small but usually profuse springs, each with its associated cluster of corn lilies—telltale indicators that water is nearby. Beyond them a steep, ducked ascent brings us up to a generally open ridge that has clusters of mountain hemlocks. From it we can look northwest down at Lake of the Woods, below us, and beyond at island-dotted Lake Aloha, which has a backdrop of the metamorphic masses of Jacks and Dicks peaks. Pyramid Peak is the prominent granitic guardian above Aloha's southwest shore.

From this ridge the trail descends a short, steep north slope to a small, boggy meadow, then makes a 1½-mile crest course north to a junction with the Lake of the Woods Trail. You, however, don't descend to the meadow, but rather follow the ridge above it briefly eastward to Ralston Peak's northwest-descending ridge. On it you may locate a faint, ducked tread, which you take southeast up to the ice-fractured quartz-monzonite summit rocks of **Ralston Peak**. At its foot lie Tamarack, Ralston, and Cagwin lakes, and to their east and below them lie Upper and Lower Echo lakes. Above the canyon beyond them are the granitic summits of the mostly unglaciated Freel Peak massif, the closest and tallest peak being 10,881-foot Freel Peak.

Perhaps the most instructive view from the summit is one north toward Fallen Leaf Lake, barely visible, and Lake Tahoe, immediately beyond it. Our view is framed by the metamorphic mass of Mt. Tallac, on the left, and the granitic mass of Echo Peak, on the right. From our vantage point, the lower southeast slope of Mt. Tallac *appears* to be almost level, and it forms a conspicuous bench from which canyon walls drop steeply to Fallen Leaf Lake. Conventional wisdom has it that the deep canyon between the two peaks was carved by glaciers. Actually, in resistant rock, which abounds in our guidebook's area, glaciers are virtually impotent at deeply eroding the landscape. However, during the last 2 million years of repeated glaciation, rockfall has been much greater than in earlier times, and the glaciers have transported a tremendous amount of rockfall debris. This has accumulated in places to form giant lateral moraines. But the amount of debris in any moraine is considerably less than one might expect, since granitic bedrock ridges lie just beneath the deposits, and they make up most of the volume of these landforms.

From Ralston Peak one can hike ½ mile southeast crosscountry quite easily along a ridge for a view down at Cup Lake, which, unlike any other lake in our area, sits in a deep hole. Could glaciers excavate such a small, deep hole? Ralston's southern slopes are, at best, minimally glaciated. Perhaps the circular basin is a meteorite-impact crater. It is the same diameter as a 140-foot-deep impact crater 2½ miles southeast from and above Lower Twin Lake (south of Bridgeport). You decide. Is there glacial evidence (moraine, polish, striations) or is there meteorite evidence (impact-fractured rock)?

Pacific Crest Trail to Lake Aloha
HIKE 10

Maps
6 and 5

Distances
3.8 miles to Tamarack Lake
4.1 miles to Ralston and Cagwin lakes
4.2 miles to Triangle Lake (via northbound trail)
5.1 miles to Echo Peak (via northbound trail)
5.1 miles to Lake Margery
5.2 miles to Lake Lucille
5.3 miles to Lake of the Woods
5.5 miles to Triangle Lake (via eastbound trail)
5.8 miles to Lake Aloha, southeast corner
6.1 miles to Lake Aloha, east shore
6.4 miles to Echo Peak (via eastbound trail)
6.7 miles to Lake LeConte
6.9 miles to Ralston Peak
7.0 miles to Ropi Lake
7.5 miles to Lake Aloha, northeast corner
9.3 miles to Clyde Lake

Directions to trailhead

From the Highway 49 junction in Placerville, drive 5 miles east up Highway 50 to the Eldorado National Forest Information Center, located on Camino Heights Drive. Get your wilderness permit there, then continue 41 miles up to Johnson Pass Road. (Westbound drivers: this road is 1¼ miles west from Echo Summit.) This road climbs 0.6 mile east to a junction, where you turn sharply left and take the Echo Lakes Road 0.9 mile north to a large parking area, most of it on the south side of the road. Park here, *not* down at Echo Lake Resort. The southbound Pacific Crest Trail starts from the smaller north part of the parking area. The northbound trail starts from Lower Echo Lake's dam, where day users usually can get wilderness permits. To reach this north trailhead, take a short steep trail northwest down to it, starting from the west end of the north part of the parking area.

Introduction

The trail from Lower Echo Lake to Lake Aloha may be the most heavily used one in the wilderness. Its popularity is due in part to its accessibility—just off Highway 50—to nearby summer homes and summer camps, and to the trail's relative ease. At 7420 feet the trailhead is about 800 feet higher than other wilderness trailheads, hence the hiker has that much less elevation to gain. Also, hikers who take the Echo Lakes water taxi can subtract 2½ miles from the above mileages. Hence only Clyde Lake, beyond Mosquito Pass, is more than 5¼ miles (or a couple of hours) away. And there are a dozen lakes that can be reached by easy cross-country hiking. No wonder the Echo Lake trailhead is so busy.

Route description

To save 5.0 miles of round-trip hiking, take the Echo Lakes water taxi, operated by Echo Lake Resort. Since Pacific Gas and Electric Company owns the top 12 feet of the lake (because they've dammed it that high), they can lower the water by that amount, and by mid-September they usually do so. Then the lake reverts to its natural, upper-lower pair of lakes, and the taxi goes only to the peninsula separating the two lakes. You'll still save 3.4 miles, round trip. The first part of Hike 10 is on a minuscule segment of the 2650-mile Pacific Crest Trail, which extends from the Canadian border to the Mexican border. This PCT segment also coincides with the Tahoe-Yosemite Trail, or TYT, the two diverging just north of Middle Velma Lake (Hike 11). This PCT segment also coincides with the Tahoe Rim Trail, or TRT, which clockwise around the Lake Tahoe Basin first follows the Big Meadow Trail south (Hike 30), the PCT north to Echo Pass (Hike 30 and, in reverse, Hike 27), then our Hike 10, and finally Hike 11 (and beyond).

We begin by crossing Lower Echo Lake's dam, make an initial climb east, and then head west on a sparsely treed, roller-coaster trail. The trail, traversing across glacier smoothed and polished lower slopes, soon takes us below some granodiorite cliffs. These and others above the Echo Lakes offer climbers about 100 routes, almost all imaginably difficult for the non-climber. In about 1 mile, at a spot below Flagpole Peak and its prominent cliffs, the trail makes a short switchback east and then climbs west high above lakeshore summer homes. Scattered Jeffrey pines and junipers give way to thick groves of lodgepoles as we descend toward the lower lake's northwest shore. We then traverse to a rusty, granitic knoll, round it to forested slopes above Upper Echo Lake, and continue westward. The tree cover is thick enough to blot out any possible view of the public pier at which the water taxis land, and use trails down to the lake may add to the confusion. If you've taken the taxi, you'll know which trail to take back. The proper trail should be signed, and it descends 120 yards to a pier. There is a nearby *pay* phone about 20 yards west of the pier, and from it you can phone the resort (659-7207) if you want a boat ride back.

Beyond the pier's trail you climb, in 0.6 mile, a rocky tread up open slopes of quartz monzonite to reach the signed Desolation Wilderness boundary and, just 15 yards past it, a junction with a trail signed for **Triangle Lake**. This is the fast way to the lake, climbing steeply ¾ mile north to a saddle, then descending ⅓ mile to the lake. If unsigned, this trail can be easily missed. It begins just 20 yards past a small bend that has conspicuous junipers growing on it and 70 yards before you enter an obvious, small grove of lodgepole pines. This route also provides the shortest way to **Echo Peak**, described below. The dark inclusions you've been seeing in the rocks over the last stretch are blocks of rock that were broken off and incorporated into rising magma that later solidified to form a pluton.

Onward, we ascend 0.6 mile past the Triangle Lake lateral, then our trail rounds a bend, passes through a dynamited, 5-foot-high trail cut, and in 40 yards reaches an obvious trail junction. From here the PCT continues to climb, while a ducked trail descends south over barren bedrock to **Tamarack Lake**, largest of the Ralston Peak basin lakes and, like the other two, fringed with mountain hemlock and lodgepole and western white pine. From the south tip of this lake you can either head south on a ducked route directly over a low ridge and descend to the north shore of moderately deep **Cagwin Lake**, lined with red mountain heather and Labrador tea, or you can follow a primitive trail southwest over the west end of the ridge and down to deep **Ralston Lake**, which is totally surrounded by steep slopes. Because these three lakes are so close to the trailhead, they are heavily used, and the Forest Service prohibits camping at them.

From the Ralston Peak basin trail junction, continue a moderate climb west up the Pacific Crest Trail to a tiny creek in a gully, then follow two switchbacks up to trail junction on a bedrock bench. From here a lateral trail traverses east across a slope predominantly colored with paintbrush and sagebrush. To reach Triangle Lake by a nearly effortless route, take this trail. On it you pass occasional junipers and view the changing perspective of the Ralston Peak basin lakes below and the peak above. Then make a

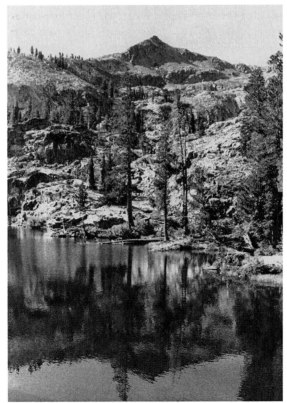

Ralston Peak reflected in Ralston Lake

brief climb to a ridge and a new panorama suddenly appears. To the east you get an aerial view of both Echo Lakes and the Sierra beyond; to the west looms Pyramid Peak above Haypress Meadows; to the south you have a detailed inspection of the basin lakes below you; and to the north you even see a bit of Lake Tahoe beyond Angora Peak. Most of the crest of the Crystal Range, northwest to around Rockbound Pass, is visible in one sweeping glance. After you have taken in this grand panorama, continue onward, descending ⅓ mile to a broad, flat saddle, where you intersect the northbound Triangle Lake trail you had met earlier.

Take this trail northward, first through a meadow then across ducked quartz-monzonite bedrock above the lake, and have an excellent view of Mt. Tallac and its southern slopes. The trail then makes a steep, 40-yard descent east. From the top of this descent, one could make an undulating traverse ⅓ mile northwest to Lost Lake, one of three lakes in our area. Lost Lake is not that appealing, however, being relatively shallow, with only cramped camping space; when the author visited it in the middle of the week—a time when the Desolation Wilderness population is vastly diminished—there were nevertheless several campers present, so don't even expect solitude. Most hikers will opt for the more appealing Triangle Lake.

From the bottom of the short, steep descent, you reach a creeklet and follow a duff trail down to the shallow, grassy south end of **Triangle Lake**. From the lake's northwest shore one can look down into the water and see brook trout swimming lazily in this deep arm of the slightly cloudy lake. Small, fair campsites can be found in nooks among the ice-fractured rocks above the lake.

Those who want to climb **Echo Peak**, 1.3 miles east of the flat saddle above Triangle Lake, follow a trail about 85 yards east-northeast to where it turns left, northeast. From there an unofficial use trail starts east (see Hike 13 for a Route description up it).

Hikers bound for Lake of the Woods, Lake Aloha, and other destinations continue along the Pacific Crest/Tahoe-Yosemite trail, leaving the junction with the eastbound trail toward Triangle Lake. Just ⅓ mile past that junction you meet the Lake of the Woods Trail, branching left to quickly pass through flowery Haypress Meadows, then climb to a proximal crest intersection of the Ralston Peak Trail. Hikers bound for **Ralston Peak** can take this trail 1⅓ miles south to a boggy meadow, and then, from a ridge just beyond it, climb ⅔ mile to the peak's summit (see Hike 9). A much closer summit from your vicinity is Keiths Dome, reached by a cross-country hike, with a 200-foot elevation gain,

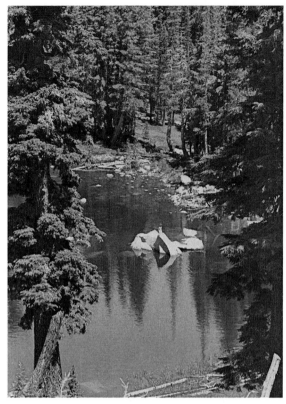

Lake Margery

north from Haypress Meadows. This easy ascent, about ½ mile long, provides you with surprisingly fine views. From the top, you could first descend southwest and then curve northwest to Lake Lucille, a more pleasant place than Lost and Triangle lakes.

Most hikers prefer to skip Ralston Peak and descend west from the crest intersection, arriving at the northeast shore of popular **Lake of the Woods** in 0.4 mile. Campsites almost girdle the lake, threatening to choke its essence. Camp at least 100 feet away from the shoreline, preferably double that. The best sites are above the west shore. From the lake's south end a trail descends 1.1 miles to **Ropi Lake**. This lake, other nearby lakes, and the routes to them are mentioned at the end of Hike 8. From Lake of the Woods' northwest corner, an official trail climbs toward Lake Aloha. Lest unofficial ones confuse you, the correct route climbs only 80 yards north, then angles west up to a gully, which it climbs to a nearby saddle; then it descends ¼ mile to the Lake Aloha Trail. The lake's southeast corner is just beyond.

About 300 yards past the Lake of the Woods Trail junction, our hike's main thoroughfare—the PCT— reaches the north end of the Ralston Peak Trail. This climbs 0.2 mile south to the crest intersection with the Lake of the Woods Trail. Just 150 yards farther on the PCT, we reach the ⅓-mile-long Lake Lucille Trail, forking right. This first descends 150 yards to a trailside pond, from which you can head cross-country 200 yards northwest to the east shore of shallow, rock-islanded, viewless **Lake Margery**. If you keep to the sometimes soggy trail, you'll reach **Lake Lucille** in ¼ mile. At its northwest shore you'll find a small, scenic peninsula, almost an island, which is a good meditative, relaxing spot for lunch (but is an illegal spot to camp).

After perhaps getting a view from the end of this lake down upon Fallen Leaf Lake and Lake Tahoe, you can follow the Lake Margery Trail up the northwest side of that lake's outlet creek. Pausing at this lake, you may see backpackers traversing high above it on the Pacific Crest expressway. Like Lake Lucille, **Lake Margery** has very limited camping potential if you camp a legal 100+ feet away from its shore. Before mid-August, this is one of the area's more mosquito-prone lakes, so camping is not that desirable. From mid-August on, camping is tolerable, but the lake's level may begin to drop, transforming it from a relatively warm, shallow swimming lake to an even shallower wading lake. The trail then winds westward to a junction with the PCT, at the south tip

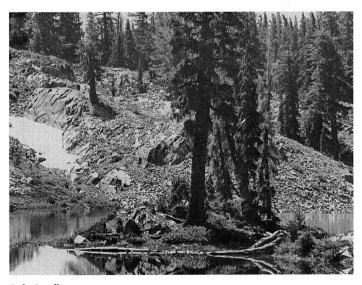

Lake Lucille

of the westernmost of three shallow, seasonal, nearly attached ponds.

If instead of visiting Lake Lucille, you keep to the PCT, you'll log just over ½ mile between the Lake Lucille and Lake Margery trail junctions. About ⅓ mile west along this stretch you'll meet the Lake Aloha Trail, which many hikers take ½ mile west down to the **south-east corner of Lake Aloha**. Approaching this corner, you'll pass the Lake of the Woods lateral—a narrow tread—about 60 yards before another lateral branches left. This one winds ¾ mile over to Lake Aloha's 20-foot-high dam, a popular swimming area when there's water in this reservoir. The great bulk of "Lake" Aloha is less than 10 feet deep, and after Labor Day the reservoir is largely emptied, creating a desolate wilderness. It is at this time that Desolation Valley's natural lakes, some up to 20 feet deep, may become revealed, as the water level drops and leaves isolated swimming holes. Lake Aloha owes its existence (and the floor of Desolation Valley owes its demise) directly to P.G.& E. and indirectly to California's ever growing population.

If you are a purist and want to adhere to the PCT all the way to Lake Aloha, then from the pond-side Lake Margery Trail junction continue northwest for 0.6 mile to another trail junction, above the **east shore of Lake Aloha**. Southward from here you can find good, legal camps between this junction and the one by the lake's southeast corner, a 0.6-mile hike south along the east-shore trail.

Over the next stretch of PCT you may see a few dead lodgepole snags, remnants of perhaps thousands that once grew in Desolation Valley before it became Lake Aloha. The lake is so shallow that when the water drops just 5 feet, you can wade across it in several places. At its height the lake is a swimmer's paradise, for then there are hundreds of bedrock islands you can reach. Should you want to swim in it, come here in the first three weeks of August, when the water is warm enough and the lake is full.

Soon our trail—the PCT or TYT, depending on your preference—takes us alongside a fairly clear, chest-deep, large pond, on our left, which like Aloha warms up to the mid-sixties in midsummer. After walking 150 yards beyond it, we reach a gully, up which our trail seems to head. A snowbank, often lasting through July, can obscure the correct route, which makes a brief climb southwest before traversing northwest again. Had you gone straight ahead on a use trail, you would have reached chilly, rockbound, trout-stocked **Lake LeConte**. This diversion would have provided you with a head-on view of towering, 9856-foot Jacks Peak.

Continuing northwest just above Lake Aloha, we now traverse along a nicer, snag-free section of the reservoir, and then reach its northeast corner, which has a two-foot-high retaining wall to prevent the lake from spilling over into Heather Lake, below us to the east. Climbing just a few yards beyond the wall, we reach a junction, from where the PCT/TYT descends first north and then east to Heather Lake. Here, at the **northeast corner of Lake Aloha**, Hike 10 ends. Hike 11 continues the PCT description through the north part of the wilderness and miles beyond it to a major Forest Service road crossing Barker Pass.

From this junction you can take a lightly used trail 7¼ miles through Rockbound Valley to Camper Flat, a base camp for adventures in the lakebound basin above it. This route, the Rubicon River Trail, first heads ¾ mile west along the north shore of Lake Aloha, providing additional water sports before you climb ¼ mile to broad, hemlock-cloaked, often snowy Mosquito Pass. It then drops a little over ½ mile to a ¼-mile-long trail that descends steeply west to **Clyde Lake**. Nestled in a cirque at the head of the Rubicon River canyon, this lake typically stays snow-lined well into August. It lacks first-class campsites, but on the other hand does provide solitude and often an ample supply of trout.

Just ⅓ mile north down the Rubicon River Trail, from the Clyde Lake spur, another spur branches 100 yards east to swampy Jacks Meadow. You then descend about one mile north to a Rubicon River ford, which has nearby camping, and along an easy grade you descend an equal distance to a second ford, with camping possibilities. You quickly reach China Flat, a meadow, then just north of it reach China Flat Public Camp, among lodgepoles and adjacent to a long, broad swimming lake. Almost ¼ mile later you ford the Rubicon for a third time. Only 300 yards past it you meet a trail that climbs 1½ miles to a junction just below Lake Doris. From that lake you can follow the reverse of the first half of Hike 7 out to Wrights Lake, about 20 miles from your starting point.

You can also continue 2⅓ miles down glaciated Rockbound Valley, passing one lateral to Lake Schmidell before reaching a second at the southern outskirts of Camper Flat. This lateral, the Blakely Trail, is just 100 yards past a trail that crosses the adjacent Rubicon River and then climbs 2¼ miles east to Middle Velma Lake. See the second half of Hike 7 for the lakes above Camper Flat. To reach Loon Lake, about 28 miles from your starting point, follow Hike 1 in reverse.

Pacific Crest Trail to McKinney Creek OHV Staging Area

HIKE 11

Maps

6, 5, 4, 3,
1 and 2

Distances

8.2 miles to Heather Lake

9.0 miles to Susie Lake

11.2 miles to Gilmore Lake

13.3 miles to Dicks Pass

15.3 miles to Dicks Lake

15.9 miles to Fontanillis Lake

17.2 miles to Middle Velma Lake

26.1 miles to Richardson Lake

29.7 miles to McKinney Creek OHV Staging Area

Directions to trailhead

Same directions as for Hike 10, but you'll probably want to leave a shuttle vehicle at the McKinney Creek OHV (Off Highway Vehicle) Staging Area. You reach this by first leaving Highway 89 in Chambers Lodge, starting south on Road 14N34 (a.k.a. County Road 3013). This road leaves Highway 89 about 1.5 miles northwest of the General Creek Campground entrance (Hike 24) and 0.1 mile east of a bridge over McKinney Creek. Follow Road 14N34 2.1 miles to McKinney Creek, then 0.2 more to the signed staging area. If you have a 4WD vehicle, you can continue 2.6 miles west to a junction, then take a jeep road 1.0 mile up to Richardson Lake.

Introduction

The first 18.5 miles of this hike's Pacific Crest Trail coincide with those of the Tahoe-Yosemite Trail. Along this popular stretch you'll see at least a dozen lakes and you'll crest the highest trail pass in Desolation Wilderness, 9380-foot Dicks Pass. This guidebook has only one trail higher, the one to 9735-foot Mt. Tallac, which is an excellent side trip easily made from this hike's Gilmore Lake.

Route description

Hike 10 describes a 7.5-mile segment of the Pacific Crest/Tahoe-Yosemite trail from Lower Echo Lake to the northeast corner of Lake Aloha. Here a retaining wall at this corner prevents the large, shallow reservoir from overflowing down to Heather Lake. The PCT leaves the west end of the wall and descends east, giving us views of the 2-mile-high Freel Peak massive to the east. A switchback takes us to a delicate 20-foot-high waterfall just above deep Heather Lake's northwest shore, and then near a large red fir and the fall's wildflower-bordered creek we find an adequate campsite.

Not much heather is found around **Heather Lake**; instead you'll see alder, dogwood, willow, and aspen, all dwarfed by the long, cold winters. The parts of bushes remaining buried and protected within the winter snow survive; parts protruding above it are likely to be killed by the icy winds. This subalpine lake is stocked with trout, but being relatively close to a popular trailhead—as all the lakes we'll pass are—catching a sizable trout may be difficult due to the high angler pressure. Most of the lakes in the wilderness have islands, but none has an island as high as the chunky, massive one in Heather Lake, which has stoutly resisted glacial attempts to wear it down.

As we traverse east above the lake's north shore, we can glance back over the lake and see ragged Pyramid Peak crowning the southern end of the Crystal Range. Our trail then leaves the lake at its check dam, climbs a low, barren ridge, and descends to a cove on the southwest shore of **Susie Lake**. In the late 1800s, routes to this and other lakes were blazed by Nathan Gilmore, discoverer of Glen Alpine Springs, and this lake was named after his oldest daughter. Given the abundance of white and red mountain heather on this shore, one might wonder if this originally was Heather Lake and Heather was Susie.

On a weekend several dozen backpackers may be seen camped at poor, tiny sites along this easily accessible, dark-shored lake below the towering, rusty, metamorphic shoulder of Jacks Peak. The best campsites are on a small bench, shaded by mountain hemlock and lodgepole pine, 70 yards down the lake's outlet creek. We cross the outlet creek, follow the rocky trail over a low ridge, pass two stagnant ponds, and descend to a flowery, swampy meadow, where the trail forks. A well-used trail to the Fallen Leaf Lake area branches southeast across the meadow (see Hike 15).

The PCT is now all uphill to Dicks Pass, and it first switchbacks northeast up to a junction with a second trail southeast down to the Fallen Leaf Lake area. This trail also continues northwest to Half Moon and Alta Morris lakes (see Hike 16). Beyond this trail intersection the PCT switchbacks up to a junction with a lateral trail that takes you 1¼ mile to good campsites above the south and east shores of orbicular **Gilmore Lake**, then 1¼ miles farther to the top of Mt. Tallac (see Hike 17).

As we start west up toward Dicks Pass, we get a peek through the lodgepole forest at Gilmore Lake, and then we ascend steadily northwest, climbing high above the pale brown metamorphic-rock basin that holds Half Moon and Alta Morris lakes. Below them to the southeast is Susie Lake, also cradled in a bed of metamorphic rock, and beyond the ridge above it we barely see Lake Aloha, nestled at the foot of Pyramid Peak and the Crystal Range. Partway up our ascent we parallel a rocky lateral moraine on our left, composed of rocks that fell onto the side of a glacier that once filled the bowl beneath us to about this height.

Our climb is enhanced by a large variety of wildflowers, and lupine, sagebrush, and juniper add pleasant aromas to the rarified air. In a rainstorm, the strong, delicious odor of wild parsley makes this small, often overlooked wildflower very noticeable. Lodgepole, hemlock, and western white pine are soon joined by whitebark pine, the harbinger of timberline, as we approach a saddle east of Dicks Peak. From it, a faint but popular unofficial trail leads hikers up a ridge to the rusty peak's summit.

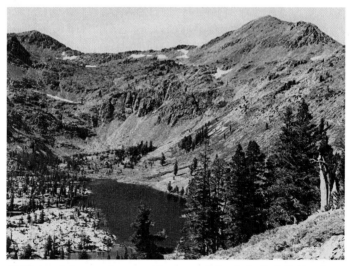

Half Moon Lake spreads out in a deep cirque below Jacks Peak (left) and Dicks Peak (right)

Rather than descend from the saddle, our trail climbs east up alongside the ridgecrest in order to bypass the steep slopes and long-lasting snowfields that lie north of it. At 9380 feet elevation our trail reaches **Dicks Pass**, an almost level area on the ridge, having clusters of dwarfed, wind-trimmed conifers and snow patches that last well into summer. Here, on the highest pass in Desolation Wilderness—and also the highest pass on the Pacific Crest Trail between Ebbetts Pass on State Highway 4 and the Canadian border, we get far-ranging views both north and south. Dicks Lake, immediately northwest below us, and Fontanillis Lake, just beyond it, are our next goals.

Ducks guide us across Dicks Pass, the boundary between metamorphic rocks to the south and granitic rocks to the north, and then we descend on hemlock-lined switchbacks, rich in thick gravel from the deeply weathered, unglaciated granodiorite bedrock. We descend northwest to a rocky saddle with sparse lodgepoles. From a junction here a trail first descends north, then traverses northeast, branching to provide two exits to the Emerald Bay area (Hikes 19 and 20). From here the PCT descends 14 miles southwest to a spur trail, which in turn descends 100 yards to a shoreline trail that leads you to campsites along the north shore and east peninsula of **Dicks Lake**.

Onward, we follow the PCT down to a large pond with a good campsite by a low ridge that blocks our view of **Fontanillis Lake**, immediately beyond it. We pass another pond before we descend a gully to a small cove on the lake's east shore and parallel this shore northwest to the outlet creek. For legal campsites look on the relatively spacious, open bedrock benches above the lake's western and southern shores.

To leave this rockbound lake, cross its outlet creek, make a brief climb north to a shady, young lateral moraine, and then descend part way along its crest before curving left, jumping an intermorainal creek and descending a slightly older lateral moraine to a trail junction above the south shore of Middle Velma Lake. Eastward, a trail climbs and then descends to Bay View Campground and to Eagle Falls Picnic Area, both above Lake Tahoe's Emerald Bay (Hikes 19 and 20).

Northwest the Velma Lakes Trail coincides with the PCT/TYT, and in about 100 yards you reach a spot where the trail bends west. Here you'll see **Middle Velma Lake**, and you can leave the trail for a quick descent to it. Its campsites are among the best you'll find along the entire route. On weekends this lakeshore is crowded, since it is quite accessible from Emerald Bay. Hikers also are attracted to its several inviting bedrock-slab islands that tempt one to swim out to, dive from, or sunbathe on them. Situated on a granitic flat between Upper and Lower Velma lakes, it drains west into the Rubicon River, whose waters eventually reach the Pacific Ocean. The other two lakes drain into Lake Tahoe, whose waters eventually reach Pyramid Lake in northwestern Nevada. A future glacial episode could alter the drainage pattern, so that Middle Velma drained east into Tahoe or Upper Velma drained northwest into the Rubicon. Only Lower Velma is set in her ways.

After climbing from the south shore back up to the PCT, we follow it ¼ mile west and reach, just 35 yards beyond a sluggish creek, a junction from which the west half of the Velma Lakes Trail descends 2¼ miles to the Rubicon River's Camper Flat. In ½ mile this lightly used trail first passes three stagnant ponds in a viewless, mosquito-prone area, then over the next ½ mile descends across slightly drier terrain. The slopes gradually steepen and the forest thins, and ½ mile later, where the trail jogs from northwest to southeast, a short spur trail departs north to a small, seasonal pool at the base of a rock slab. Onward, the descent becomes ducked as it winds down open, granitic slabs that offer views up and down the Rubicon's Rockbound Valley. Forest shade returns before you reach the valley's floor in Camper Flat. See Hikes 1, 7, and 9 for trails going, respectively, north, west, and south from this flat.

Our Hike 11 does not take this lateral, but instead adheres to the PCT/TYT. It descends briefly north to the southwest arm of Middle Velma Lake, negotiates a sometimes muddy traverse across its swampy outlet, and heads north to an abrupt change in gradient and direction. On a ¾-mile stretch we first start east and then soon curve northwest for a climb to an important junction. Here the TYT, which has coincided with the PCT, forks northwest and makes long switchbacks up to Phipps Pass. For a description along this lake-blessed, 12-mile segment to Meeks Bay, follow Hike 23 in reverse.

Our PCT forks northwest, briefly ascends a shallow gully to an almost imperceptible spur ridge, and then makes a long, gentle-to-moderate descent to seasonal Phipps Creek. Because the last glacier here removed much of the former soil, many creeks and creeklets stop flowing not long after the last snow melts. Consequently, this creek and others between Middle Velma Lake and Richardson Lake may dry up in early or mid-August. On glacier-polished granodiorite slabs just north of Phipps Creek you can find campsites that are relatively mosquito-free. After a ½-mile moderate climb north from the creek, we traverse northwest to a nearby

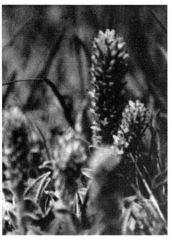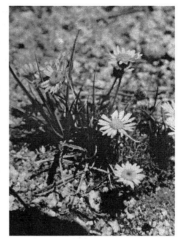

Alpine willow   *Cut-leaved daisy*

creeklet, which flows down a rock into a small pool. This has more staying power than Phipps Creek apparently because the soil on the slopes above escaped glacial erosion, and hence the creeklet is fed by groundwater. Across the creeklet we make a gentle climb to a forested spur-ridge saddle, then descend a shallow gully along the edge of a narrow meadow that runs down it. Our trail passes northeast of a 50-yard-long pond, crosses a boggy meadow beyond it, and then commences a 200-foot climb almost to the top of peak 8235.

From the PCT's local high point we can take a 40-yard spur trail southwest to some rocks, from which we can see Rubicon, Rockbound, and Buck Island reservoirs in the deep canyon west of us. A tunnel diverts water from Rubicon Reservoir to Rockbound Lake, Rockbound drains into Buck Island Lake, and a tunnel from it transports the water west, through the north end of the Crystal Range to Loon Lake. This engineering project of the Sacramento Utility District leaves the river channel below Rubicon Reservoir quite depleted, thereby depriving Hell Hole Reservoir, a down-river project of the Placer County Water Agency, of some water. It, however, receives water from a tunnel that starts at French Meadows Reservoir, which dams the Middle Fork American River. Hell Hole Reservoir, stingy like Rubicon Reservoir, usually doesn't let much water slip out down the Rubicon, but rather tunnels it through a divide to another reservoir. And so it flows—very *unnaturally*.

From the spur-trail viewpoint the PCT descends steeply to a level, northwest-trending ridge, which we follow 14 mile through an open forest to a trail junction. From here the Lake Genevieve Trail forks right and plunges via short switchbacks 0.7 mile down to a junction beside General Creek. From there, the trail continues an easy 2.0 miles east to a junction with the TYT, which goes 4.6 miles north to its trailhead at Meeks Bay (the first part of Hike 23 in reverse). Alternatively, one could take a longer trail out to Lake Tahoe, descending 1.7 miles north along General Creek, then 0.6 mile east, ending with a short climb up a road to Lost and Duck lakes. From a minor spur ridge above the creek, follow Hike 24 in reverse 5.6 miles to the trailhead at General Creek Campground, in Sugar Pine Point State Park.

The PCT veers left from the junction and in about ½ mile we have a good view before we drop into a shallow basin. We then leave it and descend a shallow gully, and after the trail levels off, one can leave it at any point for an easy, short descent west to a very open granitic bench that provides usually dry, relatively mosquito-free camping. Along this level stretch you leave Desolation Wilderness, then later, near a snow-depth indicator in a small meadow, you climb about 200 yards to a jeep-road crossing atop a forested saddle. When the last glacier was at its maximum about 20,000 years ago, it overtopped this saddle by about 80 feet, indicating that above the floor of the canyon to the west the glacier was about 1600 feet thick.

Eastbound the jeep road soon curves north, and on the PCT we parallel it on a better grade, both routes almost touching before reaching the north corner of shallow, relatively warm, 7400-foot **Richardson Lake**. At that spot we leave the Pacific Crest Trail and take the jeep road over to spacious campsites along the lake's northeast shore. Because OHVs can drive up here, you may see one or more of them at the tree-rimmed lake, especially if you arrive here on a weekend after mid-July, when the snow typically has melted.

To conclude our route, from the lake's outlet you take a jeep road northeast, then finally head east, descending a total of ¾ mile to a junction with a closed, southeast-bound road that crosses private land along its way to General Creek. You head ¼ mile north to a main OHV road, midway along this walk crossing Miller Lake's seasonal outlet, which drains west into an adjacent, waist-deep, oversize water-lily pond. You start east for a 2.6-mile trek on the main OHV road—the McKinney-Rubicon Springs jeep road. First you traverse east above Miller Lake, which is deep enough for swimming. Just beyond the east end of the lake your road crosses a creeklet feeding it, and between that and nearby, appropriately named Lily Lake, you make a barely perceptible crossing of the Sierra crest. Like the three Velma Lakes, the three lakes here empty in opposite directions, and a future glaciation could redirect Miller Lake's flow eastward. Beyond Lily Lake your road eventually passes high above the north shore of McKinney Lake, which also is an oversize water-lily pond, then it descends to your northern trailhead, the quite obvious **McKinney Creek OHV Staging Area.**

Angora Fire Lookout and Angora Lakes

HIKE 12

Maps
4 or 6

Distances
0.5 mile to Lower Angora Lake (from Angora Lakes parking lot)

0.8 mile to Upper Angora Lake (from Angora Lakes parking lot)

0.9 mile to Angora Lookout (via Clark Trail)

1.4 miles to Lower Angora Lake (via Angora Lakes Trail)

1.7 miles to Upper Angora Lake (via Angora Lakes Trail)

Directions to trailhead

From the South Lake Tahoe **Y**, where Highway 50 branches northeast toward Nevada, drive 3.1 miles on Highway 89 to Fallen Leaf Road, on the left. Take it south past Fallen Leaf Campground and, 2.0 miles from the highway, reach the north end of Tahoe Mountain Road. Drive 0.4 mile southeast up it to a junction. (This junction is also reached from the South Lake Tahoe **Y** by first driving 2.5 miles southwest on Lake Tahoe Boulevard, then driving 1.4 miles north up Tahoe Mountain Road.) From the junction drive 1.8 miles south up Angora Ridge Road 12N14 to Angora Lookout, then continue 1.0 mile to the Angora Lakes parking area. For the shortest hike to the Angora Lakes start from here.

To reach the start of the Angora Lakes Trail, take Fallen Leaf Road 4.5 miles from its Highway 89 junction to Fallen Leaf, mostly a cluster of homes at the lake's south end. Here the main road turns left, south, to climb through the complex. On it you immediately reach a short spur road branching left, east. At the end of this private road—*with no parking*—is the start of the Clark Trail. Onward, the main road curves over to a road that immediately bridges Glen Alpine Creek on its way to Stanford Sierra Camp. The Angora Lakes Trail begins south, opposite this road junction, past the east side of a chapel. The northeast corner of this junction may have enough space for a car or two. If you can't find parking by the trailhead, you can find several small turnouts along the main road, starting about 100 yards west of the trailhead.

Introduction

Since both the Clark Trail and the Angora Lakes Trail are almost exclusively used by local residents, their guests, and guests of the Stanford Sierra Camp, *neither trail is described*, although their mileages are given. The vast majority of Angora Lakes visitors take the shortest route, that is, from the Angora Lakes parking area. Be aware that even on summer weekdays (forget about weekends!) this parking area can be overflowing, so you might plan to start by midmorning, not in the afternoon. The lower lake has some cabins around it and is not heavily visited, in contrast to the upper lake, which has a resort, food and beverages, water-craft rentals, and a rather expansive beach, ideal on hot summer days for sunbathing.

Route description

To reach the Angora Lakes, merely hike up a gated road starting from the south end of the parking area. Up it you climb moderately to **Lower Angora Lake**, with private cabins, then continue on the road to **Upper Angora Lake**. Here you can rent boats from Angora Lakes Resort, buy snacks at its small store, or bask on an adjacent, attractive beach. A lucky few actually get to stay in the resort's few rental cabins. Hikers who've brought along their fishing rods will find both lakes stocked with trout. Swimmers may traverse the talus of the east shore to reach some good diving rocks

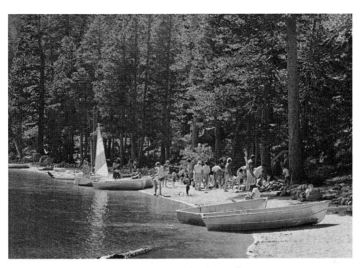

Upper Angora Lake attracts summer weekend crowds

above the south shore of this deep lake. Virtually all of our area's lakes have at least one bedrock bench from which you can dive into the lake. Here they range up to 50+ feet. However, the author cautions all would-be high divers: *do not exceed your ability*—at least one fatality has occurred, not to mention injuries. Don't let peer pressure tempt you into risky dives. An obvious diving cliff, about 15 feet high and usually with sunbathers on its sloping top, lies on the far side of the lake, and is reached by a trail along the lake's east side, by boat or raft, or by a 200-yard swim from the west end of the beach.

Returning to the parking lot, you climb to a nearby saddle, and then descend the forested Angora Lakes Trail—with several verdant oases of lush vegetation—steeply down to eventually pass the west side of a small church just before ending by a road junction with the Stanford Sierra Camp road.

Tamarack Trail to Echo Peak

HIKE 13

Maps

6

Distances

2.7 miles to Triangle Lake

3.6 miles to Echo Peak

Directions to trailhead

Hikes 13 through 17 start near Glen Alpine Creek, and since all of them enter Desolation Wilderness, you'll need a wilderness permit. The most convenient place to get one is at the Lake Tahoe Visitor Center, whose entrance is on Highway 89 about 150 yards west of Fallen Leaf Road. (This road is 3.1 miles northwest on Highway 89 from the South Lake Tahoe **Y**, where Highway 50 branches northeast from Highway 89.) With permit in hand, drive 4.5 miles south on Fallen Leaf Road, then 0.4 mile west through Fallen Leaf Lake's south-shore development to a junction with Road 12N15 branching right. This immediately bridges Glen Alpine Creek before ending at Stanford Sierra Camp. If you take the entire described route, your Hike 13 will end at the junction. However, it begins 0.4 mile farther up the main road, Road 12N16, and 300 yards before the road bridges cascading Glen Alpine Creek. Immediately beyond the bridge is the moderately large Glen Alpine trailhead parking area (for Hikes 14-17), which usually has wilderness permits for *day users.* You can also park here, if it's not full, or along small turnouts along your narrow road up to the parking area.

Introduction

The *unmaintained* Tamarack Trail is also known as the Tamarack Lake Trail, even though it does not go to Tamarack Lake. "Triangle Lake Trail" would be a better name, although "Tamarack Trail" is okay since the trail does pass a number of tamaracks, a.k.a. lodgepole pines. This lightly used trail provides a direct route to Triangle Lake that is comparable in energy expended to that in Hike 10. (That hike is easier *only* if you take the water taxi.) Additionally, you can climb to Echo Peak and then descend a use route to Upper Angora Lake, an ideal relaxing site after your arduous climb. The wildflowers along the ascent usually are so abundant that plant lovers can feel rewarded even without climbing to the lake.

Before mid-July the Tamarack Trail may be too dangerous. Hike 13's alternate descent route from Echo Peak to Upper Angora Lake is safe for cautious hikers, but is so steep that few would want to ascend it. It is, however, the shortest way to the top, only 2.0 miles from the Angora Lakes parking area (see Hike 12's "Directions to trailhead").

Route description

Starting on metamorphic bedrock with granitic boulders transported here by a glacier, the trail enters an open forest of white fir and lodgepole and Jeffrey pine, with a rich substory of aspen, alder, willow, vine maple, tobacco brush, currant, and spiraea. Beyond a low knoll we get a view of Mt. Tallac's dark back side, then enter a shady forest. Now a steep ascent begins, but thirst on this climb can be slaked at a number of refreshing creeklets, each with its own population of water-loving plants.

The grade eases and the forest opens as we approach a second knoll, from which we can look west-northwest at the two brownish-red metamorphic summits of Jacks and Dicks peaks. Near us is a huge, 20-foot-high orange-and-gray block of metamorphic rock in contact with granitic rock that intruded it about 90 million years ago. Beyond it we are soon climbing up steep switchbacks through an overwhelming amount of vegetation. Finally emerging from this jungle, we make a short traverse west to a relatively barren flat on which a few hardy junipers survive. From here we have an inspiring view of most of Fallen Leaf Lake and part of Tahoe beyond it. Now also visible is Mt. Tallac's rusty summit. Just above our flat is an exposed campsite, relatively close to a long-lasting snowfield, and both are just inside the Desolation Wilderness boundary.

For many, this is as far as they may want to ascend, because now a short, climbing traverse west brings us to a *dangerous creek* we must jump across. Should you slip, you're likely to go over the brink of a very steep cascade. Short, steep switchbacks up a path gloriously lined with wildflowers take us to a safe recrossing of the creek and to some good rocks to stop at and rest, from which one can photograph the magnificent canyon and lateral moraines to the north.

Refreshed, we climb steeply up the wildflowered east bank of the creek, cross it after a 250-foot climb, then continue up an increasingly easy grade that eventually levels off. Here we see a panorama from Lake Tahoe past Tallac, Dicks, and Jacks summits to barely showing Pyramid Peak. From this vicinity, adept hikers can start a cross-country jaunt west to Triangle Lake, saving ½ mile. Along a nearly level stretch of trail the forest now is an open one of juniper, western white pine, and mountain hemlock, and on slopes grasses, sedges, sagebrush, and drought-resistant wildflowers grow. An easy stroll next takes us down to a flat saddle with a trail intersection. To the north, the trail descends to **Triangle Lake**; south, it descends to the Echo Lakes (see Hike 10 for more details).

To climb Echo Peak, retrace your steps 85 yards east-northeast to where your trail turns left, northeast. From there you start east up an unofficial use trail. This quickly curves northeast, and one basically just ascends directly upslope. The topography and vegetation are so amenable to cross-country travel that you need not attempt to look for a trail. You climb through an open forest that now includes whitebark pine; then eventually reach the rocky northwest ridge of Echo Peak.

Here it behooves you to walk 130 yards north to the brink of the ridge, from where you not only see everything you might have seen from the Angora Lookout (Hike 12), but also have a better perspective of it all. Very conspicuous is Mt. Tallac's preglacial, almost flat erosion surface, which has remained little changed over millions of years. Glaciers eroded the deep canyon below it, but not nearly so much as glaciologists would have us believe. Dated, ancient lava flows on the slopes and floors of glaciated Sierran canyons allow one to reconstruct ancient canyons. Doing so shows that they had already attained their "glacial topography" some 30 million years before the first major glaciers ever entered them. Glaciers merely accentuated the features of the preglacial topography.

From where we reached the northwest ridge, an easy, ducked route southeast takes us to granitic, potholed **Echo Peak**, which gives us an additional panorama, one of the Crystal Range to the south and west. On the southeast horizon near Carson Pass stand Stevens and Red Lake peaks, both just over 10,000 feet in elevation. Like every other Tahoe peak, ours has its resident golden-mantled ground squirrel to inspect you or your pack, if you leave it for a minute.

Descend the way you came, or else descend to Upper Angora Lake. To do that, start east from the summit on a ducked use trail through gruss, which is an accumulation of feldspar and quartz crystals that have broken off weathered granitic rock after the dark minerals disintegrated and freed them. The use trail soon starts a descent on a very steep, minor northeast ridge of Echo Peak, and then it continues down a gully so rich in gruss that you can almost ski down it. Large backpacks are definitely not recommended on this very steep descent. Several short-switchback routes descend northeast down this gully and merge on a flat 300 feet above the lake. Midway down the very steep gully someone long ago placed a facetious sign, *Caution—Maximum Speed 25 Mi*.

From the flat, descend northwest very steeply down another gully to Upper Angora Lake's southeast corner. Here you can traverse west to a rock slab above the south shore, from which you can dive into water that is deep for a lake its size—48 feet. There is also plenty of room on the slab for those who just like to sunbathe.

The trail from the southeast corner consists of a traverse across a large-block talus slope to the lake's outlet, then a walk northwest to Angora Lakes Resort. From here follow Hike 12's description down to a trailhead on Fallen Leaf Road, then hike southwest 0.4 mile up the road to your original trailhead.

Grass Lake

HIKE 14

Maps
4 or 6

Distances
2.6 miles to Grass Lake

Directions to trailhead

See directions under Hike 13

Introduction

An easy day hike, this route leads to a rockbound lake with a dramatic cascade on the cliffs beyond it. Its fairly warm water is just right for a midsummer afternoon swim. Being so close to the trailhead, the lake has developed vegetation, sanitation, and soil problems due to overuse. Hence if you feel you absolutely must camp at Grass Lake, do so with minimum impact (no fires; carry out *all* wastes).

Route description

From the Glen Alpine trailhead parking area you walk west about 1.1 miles on a closed road past private homes to where a trail begins just beyond Glen Alpine Springs. Nathan Gilmore discovered these mineral springs—high in bicarbonate, chloride, sodium, and calcium—while looking for his stray cattle in 1863. They were then gushing at about 200 gallons an hour. In the late 1870s Gilmore began bottling the carbonated water, which soon achieved a reputation, and he developed Glen Alpine Springs into a very popular resort.

Start up the Glen Alpine Trail, which soon climbs southeast about 200 yards before climbing west up a rocky, joint-controlled gully. You make a switchback south out of the gully, curve around a low ridge, and walk west again to a small, waist-deep pool with a tiny fall splashing into it. Just beyond it, on a flat immediately before the trail bends northeast as it starts a switchbacking climb, we arrive at a junction with the Grass Lake Trail. From here, head a few yards west, jump across Gilmore Lake's outlet creek, which here is part of the Desolation Wilderness boundary, and fol-

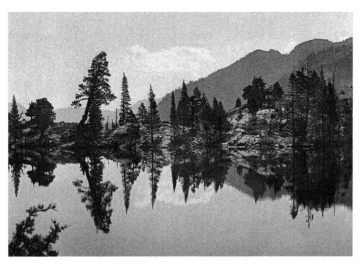

Grass Lake

low the trail southwest up a brushy slope to reach a grassy pond that is an overflow of Glen Alpine Creek. The best spot to cross this creek is at some rapids below the pond, where water flows east down a small, granitic, 20-foot-high **V** gorge.

Beyond this crossing our trail winds almost up to the out-let creek of Lake Lucille. You may see an older trail that still climbs southwest to it before curving northwest to Grass Lake, but our trail curves north, passes northwest through a **V** trough, and then curves southwest and descends through another one. Joint control certainly expresses itself in this granodiorite bedrock. Just beyond the second trough our trail meets the older trail, and 100 yards far-ther we are at the southeast corner of shallow **Grass Lake**. The trail continues 0.2 mile to a shallow bay, passing several campsites located too close to the shoreline to be legal. For legal camping, continue westward.

Lining the south shore are some metavolcanic rocks, below which is the lake's deepest water. Here, an eight-foot-high rock bench makes an ideal platform for diving into the lake's fair-ly clear water, which warms up into the mid-60s. These brown rocks contrast strongly with the gray, joint-controlled granitic ones that dam the lake's east end. Fishing is poor because the lake is rel-atively small and is heavily fished. However, what may be lost in the way of a trout dinner is compensated for by the lovely lakeside surrounding, including a silvery cascade from Susie Lake that splashes down the cliff northwest of us.

Glen Alpine to Lake Aloha

HIKE 15

Maps
4 and 3

Distances
4.1 miles to Susie Lake
5.2 miles to Heather Lake
6.1 miles to Lake Aloha

Directions to trailhead

See directions under Hike 13

Introduction

This trip takes you up to large, shallow Lake Aloha, which is probably the most popular lake in Desolation Wilderness. By arriving at its scenic northeast shore, however, you avoid most backpackers, who generally camp at its south shore. Rockbound Susie Lake, two-thirds of the way up to Aloha, is a favorite lake of many backpackers, and for late-season excursions it is a well-chosen goal, because much of Aloha dries up after Labor Day. Before then, both Susie and Heather lakes may be too crowded—at least on weekends—to suit your fancy.

Route description

As in Hike 14 start at a gate, walk 1.1 miles up a closed road, then hike up the Glen Alpine Trail to a small flat just above a splashing trailside pool. Above this flat and its Grass Lake Trail junction, you make a switchbacking ascent northward up a brushy, open-forested granitic slope, where golden-mantled ground squirrels forage about.

Beyond a step-across creeklet, we continue up the Glen Alpine Trail to Gilmore Lake's outlet creek—which one must wade in early summer—and then in 30 yards reach a trail fork. The right fork climbs to a junction with trails to Half Moon Lake, Dicks Pass, Gilmore Lake, and Mt. Tallac (Hikes 16 and 17). We take the left fork, which makes an initial climb west, traverses through a lodgepole forest past four water-lily ponds, and then descends westward to join the Pacific Crest/Tahoe-Yosemite trail. Here, at the upper end of a boggy meadow, you can identify an abundant variety of wildflowers—after mid-August, when the mosquitoes aren't pestering you to death. Identified by their aromas are swamp onion, lupine, and coyote mint. Also look for tiger lily, corn lily, buttercup, columbine, ligusticum, paintbrush, senecio, yarrow, and daisy.

From the junction our route follows the PCT/TYT west past **Susie Lake** and **Heather Lake** up to **Lake Aloha**. See the first part of Hike 11 for a more complete description in reverse.

Half Moon and Alta Morris Lakes
HIKE 16

Maps
4 and 3

Distances
4.8 miles to Half Moon Lake
5.5 miles to Alta Morris Lake

Directions to trailhead

See directions under Hike 13

Introduction

Situated on the corrugated bedrock floor of an immense cirque, Half Moon and Alta Morris lakes see relatively little use despite their accessibility; they are bypassed for lakes in more demure settings along the highly popular Pacific Crest/Tahoe-Yosemite trail. Within this cirque basin you're almost guaranteed to find a suitable, isolated campsite.

Route description

Start as in Hike 15. From Gilmore Lake's outlet creek junction where Hike 15 forks left, our route forks right. We make a ¼-mile ascent up a rocky path, climbing steadily above a shallow tarn below us to a juniper-flat intersection with the Pacific Crest/Tahoe-Yosemite trail, and go straight ahead.

Our trail starts a contour northwest, then arcs west across a small, forested bowl. Leaving the bowl, we climb to a low ridge and see Susie Lake, nestled in her metamorphic bed. On the skyline, Pyramid Peak stands at the south end of a long stretch of the granitic Crystal Range. Leaving this viewpoint, we descend slightly into a shallow gully, go up it, cross a low ridge bordering it, and then traverse a lodgepole flat and a mucky-banked creeklet flowing through it. Next we climb up the southwest slope of yet another gully and soon approach a chest-deep pond, on the left. After passing two smaller ponds on the right, which support pond lilies and other aquatic vegetation, we come to a grass-lined pond with a campsite on its northeast shore. Since this site is within 100 feet of the shoreline, it is off limits, so if you want to camp in this vicinity, try above the south or west shore.

From a low ridge immediately beyond the last pond, we see clear, appropriately named **Half Moon Lake**, which occupies almost the entire width of the huge cirque lying between Jacks Peak and Dicks Pass. Not only is this the largest cirque in Desolation Wilderness, but it is also the deepest, and the lake is hemmed in on three sides by a dark wall of steep rock that averages 1300 feet high.

The trail makes an undulating traverse across a meadowy talus slope of metamorphic rock that borders the lake's north and west shores. In some places the trail is boggy; in others it is indistinct and somewhat overgrown with willows. Eventually you'll reach a fairly large campsite, nestled under pines and hemlocks, on a bench above the northwest shore of **Alta Morris Lake**. This lake, perhaps the most scenic cirque lake in the wilderness, rests above the southwest corner of Half Moon Lake, and it can be approached by a more direct, drier, cross-country route.

Starting this route when you first see Half Moon Lake, head west and stay on the rocky bench above its south shore. On Maps 4 and 3 this route looks almost level, but in reality you ascend and descend a number of small, glacier-smoothed gullies. Midway across your washboard traverse you'll cross Half Moon's outlet creek, which cascades into a clear, linear, grassy-bottomed lakelet that is nice to camp near. Continuing west toward the dark rusty-brown metamorphosed sandstone-and-mudstone east buttress of Jacks Peak, you walk across buff-colored metamorphosed conglomerate that contrasts strongly with it. Soon you reach one or more small, semistagnant ponds and, just beyond them, the northeast bench above Alta Morris Lake. Trout fishing, hopefully, will be good at both lakes.

Mt. Tallac via Gilmore Lake
HIKE 17

Maps
4

Distances
4.2 miles to Gilmore Lake
6.0 miles to Mt. Tallac

Directions to trailhead
See directions under Hike 13

Introduction
Of all the significant peaks you can climb by trail, Mt. Tallac is the closest one to Lake Tahoe's shore. Consequently, your lake view is truly exceptional, and it is highlighted by the dramatic, linear, prodigious lateral moraines that border Emerald Bay, Cascade Lake, and Fallen Leaf Lake. Gilmore Lake, along your ascent route, is an ideal spot to rest or camp before making the final push for the summit.

Route description
Follow Hike 15 up to Gilmore Lake's outlet creek junction, fork right, and climb to the juniper-flat Pacific Crest/Tahoe-Yosemite trail junction. From here Hike 16 continues straight ahead to Half Moon and Alta Morris lakes, but your route switchbacks north up a ½-mile piece of the PCT/TYT. Along this open ascent past large, rusty-barked junipers, you can look south to shallow Grass Lake and southwest to sparsely tree-lined Susie Lake.

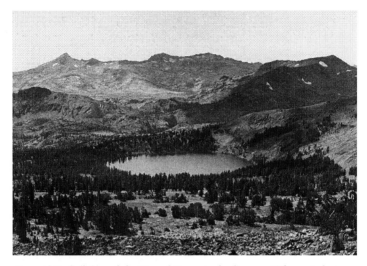

Pyramid Peak (left) and the Crystal Range in the distance, Gilmore Lake in the foreground

Just before the trail comes alongside Gilmore Lake's cascading outlet creek, you catch a glimpse of granite-lined Lake Aloha in the southwest. Veering slightly away from the creek, you reach an almost level junction in an open lodgepole forest.

The PCT/TYT turns west and continues its climb to Dicks Pass (see Hike 11), but we head north, cross the creek and arrive at the southeast shore of **Gilmore Lake**. In the entire Sierra there is hardly a lake more circular than this one, and it is amazing that it doesn't bear the name *Round Lake*, especially when you consider how many noncircular lakes in the Sierra do bear this name. Instead, it was named in honor of Nathan Gilmore, a local settler from 1863 onward, who in 1877 stocked this lake with 20 black bass. Now it has a population of trout, like other lakes. Please don't camp at the lake's overused southeast shore; rather, use fine, lodgepole-shaded campsites above the lake's south and east shores.

Beyond this lake our trail climbs steeply, first northeast and then north, heading up through a rapidly thinning forest of lodgepole and whitebark pines and crossing three flower-lined creeklets. We hike to within 150 yards of a 9000-foot saddle, then switchback east up the grass- and sagebrush-lined trail. About 200 feet below the summit we reach a junction with the Mt. Tallac Trail, which descends Tallac's southeast slope and then curves north down toward Highway 89. Hike 18 describes the route from this junction to the summit of **Mt. Tallac**, the views seen from it, and the significant geomorphic features.

Mt. Tallac via Floating Island Lake
HIKE 18

Maps	*Distances*
4	1.7 miles to Floating Island Lake
	2.5 miles to Cathedral Lake
	4.6 miles to Mt. Tallac

Directions to trailhead

From where Highway 50 leaves Highway 89 in South Lake Tahoe, drive 3.2 miles northwest on Highway 89 to the Lake Tahoe Visitor Center, whose entrance is just 150 yards west of Fallen Leaf Road. If you're going to Floating Island Lake or beyond, get a wilderness permit here (they usually are also available, *for day hikers only*, at the trailhead). Westward, you bridge Taylor Creek in ¼ mile, then in another ½ mile reach a signed intersection. From here most folks drive ½ mile north to Baldwin Beach, but on a paved road you head south, branching left in 0.4 mile, then keeping right at a quickly reached second fork. You then drive _ mile to a parking area with space for at least a dozen vehicles. This trailhead usually has wilderness permits for *day users*.

Introduction

Like Hike 17, this one takes you to Mt. Tallac's summit, but it does so in fewer miles. Two small lakes—one of them unique—are passed along your way up this route, which has more views but fewer campsites than does Hike 17. Hence it is best done as a day hike.

Route description

You start among Jeffrey pines and sagebrush, climb 120 yards up an old road to a blocked-off fork, veer right, and reach an old gravel pit. The gap here offers a glimpse of the structure of a glacial moraine, which is largely composed of unsorted boulders in a gravel matrix. Beyond the pit we're now on a trail, climbing south up a shallow gully that lies between two lateral moraines. The east one was left by the last glacier to occupy the basin now filled by Fallen Leaf Lake. The west one probably was deposited by the same glacier, earlier in its history. A larger, unseen moraine lies west of it, this one terminating at about the 6400-foot elevation, just south of the major bend in Highway 89. We'll be crossing that moraine near Floating Island Lake.

Starting toward that lake, we make a moderate climb south, the gradient rapidly reducing to gentle. In ⅓ mile we crest the moraine, which is largely cloaked in huckleberry oaks and greenleaf manzanitas on its east slopes and in white firs and Jeffrey pines on its west slopes. Our first views are stunning, but better ones lie ahead as we traverse south. After a ½-mile walk we drop away from the crest, being saturated with views of Fallen Leaf Lake, Lake Tahoe, and the Freel Peak massif. We enter another intermorainal gully, then make a rocky ascent across the earlier moraine, the ascent yielding to a brief traverse into a red-fir forest. Under deep shade we make a short, steep climb south up almost useless switchbacks, then level off just inside the Desolation Wilderness boundary by the north end of shallow **Floating Island Lake**.

In 1890 this unique lake was noted as having a 20-foot-diameter floating mat of grass and shrubs, whence the name. In more recent times there have been several floating, grassy mats, and more mats are ready to slough off from the lake's soggy northwest shore. It's a mystery why mats slough off at this lake and not at any other, for in all other respects this lake seems quite ordinary. Anyway, mats do slough off here, replacing older mats that break up. Therefore chances are very good that you'll see at least one island floating in this lake. Conifers ring this lake, denying space for a legal campsite.

Climbing toward Cathedral Lake, you leave Floating Island Lake and parallel its inlet creek to a nearby gap. From it an essentially cross-country route—formerly a trail—traverses south 0.2 mile to a trail from Fallen Leaf Lake. We head southwest up our trail, lined with wildflowers, currant, service-berry, sagebrush, and other shrubs we've seen, and soon come to a saddle immediately west of a little rocky knoll. From its juniper-covered summit, free of mosquitoes, we can relax and take in a panorama that includes most of Lake Tahoe, some of Fallen Leaf Lake, and beyond it the granitic summits of the Freel Peak massif.

Mt. Tallac's summit area is now visible, and it beckons us onward, so we make a brief descent to Cathedral Creek, cross it, and meet a trail from Fallen Leaf Lake. This descends, excessively so in one stretch, 1.0 mile to a junction about 130 feet above the

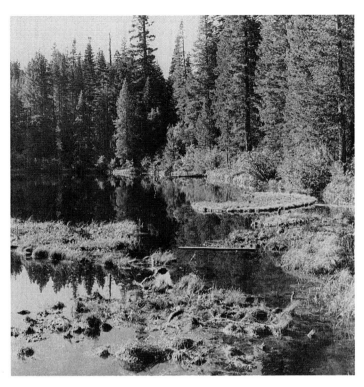

Floating Island Lake

lake's west shore. From here a trail heads ⅓ mile south to the private grounds of Stanford Sierra Camp, while in the other direction it heads ⅔ mile north to the Fallen Leaf Tract summer homes. There's hardly any space to park at this north trailhead, and the hot, steep nature of this trail to Cathedral Lake makes it the least desirable route to Mt. Tallac.

Just a few minutes' hiking past the trail from Fallen Leaf Lake, our trail from Floating Island Lake reaches **Cathedral Lake**. Named for its proximity to Cathedral Peak, which is not a peak but rather a cliff on Tallac's southeast ridge, this mostly shallow lake does support a few trout. Its water is clearer than that of Floating Island Lake, and swimming is fair along its south shore. As at the previous lake, legal campsites 100+ feet from the shore are hard to find. A path of sorts skirts the lake's west and south shores, from which one can climb a chaotic jumble of huge talus blocks for a view of the Tahoe scenery.

However, better views are at Tallac's summit, so make a very steep climb 200 feet above Cathedral Lake to a trail segment with water usually running along it. Bordered with monkey flower, stickseed, larkspur, fireweed, thimbleberry, and other hydrophytic plants, this short stretch is an excellent place to take a lunch break, since it may be your last dependable source of water. Beyond it the trail climbs steadily and steeply up the sloping floor of a cirque toward its headwall, which usually has snowfields well into August. Several trails, formed on talus through continued use, try to avoid most of the snow. The correct route has a switchback leg that climbs *south* up to the top. Once on it we have great views east, south, and west—a taste of what's to come.

We leave the edge of Tallac's southeast ridge as we hike northwest up an increasingly steep trail bordered by currant, gooseberry, snow bush, spiraea, and sagebrush. Also, clusters of western white, lodgepole, and whitebark pines speckle the slope. Near the 9000-foot level, the brush diminishes and wildflowers become more predominant. At about the 9400-foot level you may see an abandoned trail going directly downslope, leading unwary descending hikers astray. Finally, in just over 200 yards, we reach a junction with the trail from Gilmore Lake (see Hike 17). Enjoying a breather while taking in a view of the lakes and ponds below, we can identify circular Gilmore Lake in its cirque southwest of us, Susie Lake on a bench beyond it, and Lake Aloha along the east base of the granitic Crystal Range.

There being now only 200 vertical feet to climb to the summit, we first head east to a weatherbeaten clump of conifers, which makes a good wind-protected emergency shelter, but is no place to sit out a lightning storm. You should not attempt to climb to this summit—or any summit—if a storm is impending. We now follow a rocky route, first northeast to the brink of a dangerously steep avalanche chute, then diagonally northwest for the last few steps to the pointed summit. Most panoramas from any high summit are spectacular, but those from dark, metamorphic **Mt. Tallac** are exceptional. Because it stands so close to Lake Tahoe, it offers a view of almost the entire lake, and we can study the major currents that swirl about in it. Standing above Tahoe's northeast end is andesite-capped Mt. Rose, which at 10,776 feet is the basin's third highest peak. Along the east shore rise the granitic western slopes of the Carson Range, which remain unglaciated because they lie within a rain shadow cast by the Sierra crest above Tahoe's western shore. Today the western crest receives 70-90 inches of precipitation annually, whereas the eastern crest receives only about 30-40 inches.

Along the lake's south shore are the readily visible Tahoe Keys, which together with the highrises stand out in this basin as a monument to man's economic exploitation of a unique high-mountain lake basin that should have been a national park. Southeast of this shore rise 10,881-foot Freel Peak and 10,823-foot Jobs Sister, ranking first and second among the basin's peaks. In the distance to the southeast is the 10,000-foot ridge near Carson Pass. To the south rises granitic Echo Peak, and beyond it Ralston Peak, the unseen Echo Lakes lying between them. West of Ralston Peak is Pyramid Peak, the high point and south end of the Crystal Range.

Of much interest are the huge, linear, lateral moraines that border Emerald Bay, Cascade Lake, and Fallen Leaf Lake. Their crests are as much as 1100 feet above adjacent basin floors, and this relief indicates the *minimum* thickness of the glaciers that filled the basins. The Tahoe basin must have been an extremely impressive sight some 130-200,000 years ago. During that time large glaciers from Squaw Valley, and from Pole Creek north of it, periodically dammed Tahoe's outlet and raised the lake's level. And then glaciers from the Upper Truckee River canyon and from every canyon along the lake's west shore north to its outlet reached the lake, spalling icebergs into its frigid, deep water.

Granite Lake and
Cascade Creek Fall
HIKE 19

Maps
4

Distances
0.7 mile to Cascade Creek Fall
1.1 miles to Granite Lake
2.7 miles to Emerald Bay Trail

Directions to trailhead

From where Highway 50 leaves Highway 89 in South Lake Tahoe, drive 3.2 miles northwest on Highway 89 to the Lake Tahoe Visitor Center. Get your wilderness permit here—unless you're going only to Cascade Creek Fall—then continue 4.5 miles on Highway 89 to Bay View Campground, on your left. (Southbound drivers: from Tahoe City follow Highway 89 south 2.2 miles to the William Kent Visitor Center, get your wilderness permit, then continue 17½ miles to Bay View Campground. This campground is one mile southeast of Eagle Falls Picnic Area.) Drive through the campground to a parking area which holds about three dozen vehicles. Don't park in the campground's sites.

Introduction

A pleasant day hike, the Bay View Trail leads you up to lovely Granite Lake, a good lake for swimming since it is one of the Tahoe basin's warmest lakes. For those with less time on their hands, the Cascade Creek Fall Trail provides them with a fine Lake Tahoe view from the brink of a waterfall. Cascade Lake, into which Cascade Creek tumbles, is largely on private land, although one could descend to the lake's southwest shore, which is on National Forest land.

Route description

From the trailhead parking area the Cascade Creek Fall Trail branches left while the Bay View Trail starts straight ahead, and will be described first. From the trailhead you climb moderately through a dense white-fir forest with a chinquapin understory, then switchback up to a sharp bend in an old jeep road. Now you immediately enter Desolation Wilderness as you follow the closed jeep road northwest up to the top of a ridge of weathered granodiorite bedrock. By walking a few paces north, you'll obtain a tree-framed view of Emerald Bay, its bedrock Fannette Island, and Lake Tahoe.

Your route ahead is now a trail that climbs southeast alongside Granite Lake's trickling, alder-lined outlet creek. Also along it you find water-loving wildflowers, including Bolanders yampah, or olaski, as the Miwok Indians called it, who ate the roots of this wild carrot. Don't pick this plant because, first, it is illegal to do so, and second, there are some poisonous wild carrots that closely resemble it. The sensuous aroma of tobacco brush heralds our approach to moderately large **Granite Lake**. You'll appre-

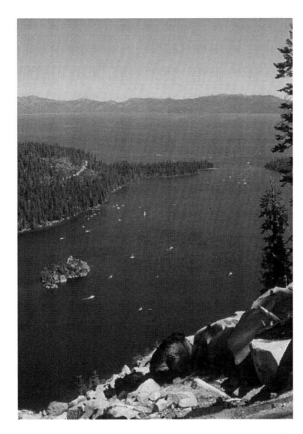

View from Bay View Trail

ciate the relatively warm water—up to 70°F—of this clear lake. A broad moraine lies at its north end, and the lake's outlet flows along bedrock beneath it. There are no large campsites, but small ones lie along its east and north shores. However, due to its proximity to Highway 89, the lake should be day-use only.

Beyond this lake the Bay View Trail climbs 1.6 miles over Maggies Peaks and down to a junction with the Emerald Bay Trail. Both trails are overly steep, but the Emerald Bay Trail to this junction is about ¼ mile shorter and has about 100 feet less elevation gain. Hikers favor that trail, while equestrians have no choice; to enter the wilderness from this general area, they are required to take our better-graded Bay View Trail. In a nutshell, this switchbacks high above Granite Lake, traverses gentle slopes below forested South Maggies Peak, then weaves a contorted ½-mile route down to a junction with the Emerald Bay Trail. See Hike 20 if you're bound for some wilderness lakes.

The other choice in our Hike 19 menu is a short excursion over to Cascade Creek Fall. Starting from the trailhead, you branch left, southeast, for a 110-yard climb to a brushy crest of a lateral moraine, then head 150 yards southwest along it. From the crest you next have a ½-mile footpath across steep slopes to the brink of the fall. Because all but the start of the path is across either brushy or rocky slopes, you have almost continual views of Cascade Lake and Lake Tahoe. Your descending, brushy traverse turns into a climb up rocky slabs, upon which the trail dies out. To reach the brink of the falls is easy, but be careful as you approach it, since a slip over the brink would certainly be fatal. This spot is a fine one for a picnic, since the views rival those from the brink of Eagle Falls, above Emerald Bay, and here you don't have the crowds.

A surprising number of backpackers head cross-country up Cascade Creek to Snow and Azure lakes, but the route is vague and it can be dangerous in spots, so it is not described here.

Velma Lakes Area
HIKE 20

Maps	**Distances**
4 and 3	1.0 mile to Eagle Lake
	4.3 miles to Dicks Lake
	4.4 miles to Middle Velma Lake
	4.5 miles to Upper Velma Lake
	4.9 miles to Fontanillis Lake (via Dicks Lake)
	5.2 miles to Fontanillis Lake (via Middle Velma Lake)

Directions to trailhead

From where Highway 50 leaves Highway 89 in South Lake Tahoe, drive 3.2 miles northwest on Highway 89 to the Lake

Tahoe Visitor Center. Get your wilderness permit here, then continue 5.6 miles on Highway 89 to the moderately large but often overflowing parking lot of Eagle Falls Picnic Area, immediately past Eagle Creek. Since the parking lot can be completely full by 10 A.M. on a summer weekday, and earlier on weekends, try to start your hike as early as possible. Be aware that there is a $3 per day parking fee. If you're driving from Tahoe City, follow Highway 89 south 2.2 miles to the William Kent Visitor Center, get your wilderness permit, and then continue 16½ miles to the picnic area. This usually has wilderness permits for *day users*. Lock your car, for thefts are all too common here.

Introduction

Despite its difficulty, the trail up Eagle Lake canyon is one of the most popular in the Tahoe region, for it takes you, in a few hours' time, to the Dicks Lake—Velma Lakes area. By making a loop through this area you pass at least five lakes and one lakelet, all good for swimming or camping.

Route description

At times incorrectly signed the Eagle Falls Trail (the falls are *east* of Highway 89), our trail makes a brushy ascent southwest up-canyon, climbs past a vertical cliff, then bridges Eagle Creek. The bridge could easily support horses and their riders, but this trail is for hikers only; equestrians must use the Bay View Trail (Hike 19), which has equestrian trailhead parking. From the bridge our footpath cuts across the base of a blocky talus slope, climbs up to a bench, and enters Desolation Wilderness as it swings west to a second bench, on which lie erratic boulders transported down-canyon by a glacier. From this bench we can look northeast down at Emerald Bay and out to the Carson Range above Tahoe. Beyond the bench we cross a small lodgepole flat, round a low headwall, and parallel Eagle Lake's outlet creek. Shortly we reach another flat, shaded by white firs and Jeffrey pines. We now make a brief ascent, see the creek's rapids, and catch a glimpse of **Eagle Lake** as we reach a well-used spur trail that goes 200 yards over the bedrock to the lake. This picturesque lake is hemmed in by granitic cliffs, which along with cliffs you passed down-canyon, attract talented rock climbers. Non-climbers will find a lake to relax at, to photograph, or to fish in.

Beyond this lake the Emerald Bay Trail climbs steeply to a saddle and a junction with the Bay View Trail. On this strenuous climb, aromatic tobacco brush, drab huckleberry oak, and needle-

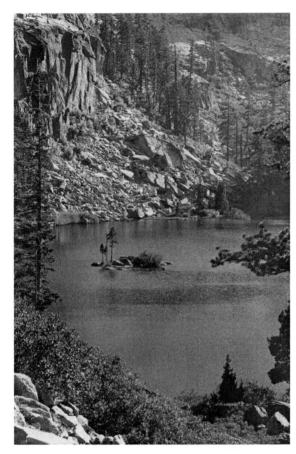

Eagle Lake

tipped snow bush dominate the vegetation. This section is a bad one for wearing shorts on or carrying a large pack up. Starting up it, we first pass under the towering cliff of North Maggies Peak, then arrive at a gully, shaded by pines and firs, that has a trickling creeklet. Short, steep switchbacks lead up the gully's west side and higher up we arrive at a barren slab leading to a small flat with lodgepole pines. Our trail traverses its west side for 50 yards before climbing south-southwest up to and through a clump of alders, arriving at the base of an outcrop. After an initial 30-yard climb west along this base our trail, which can be indistinct over the last ¼ mile, becomes obvious, and we climb south steeply up a slope and then traverse to a rocky bench on the west ridge of South Maggies Peak. These two similar, pointed peaks, popular conversation for 19th century Lake Tahoe boaters, were named not for Maggie but for her breasts. Back in those days, the two peaks' names were more explicit. (Today, Wyoming's Grand Teton survives unchanged because the name is French, and therefore not offensive.)

A short, steep switchback leg takes us down from the bench, and then we make a traverse high above a large pond overgrown with grass and pond lilies. Along the trail we find, in an alder thicket, a trickling spring, which is the last dependable water until Velma Lakes creek, about 2 miles ahead. Beyond the spring we switchback up to an ephemeral creek, cross it, and climb a gradually easing slope to a saddle on which we meet the Bay View Trail. From here we traverse west, pass two ridgetop ponds, and then make a ½-mile traverse past brush and bedrock almost to a saddle. Here, near a small, seasonal, ankle-deep pond, is a junction.

From it the trail to Dicks Lake traverses ½ mile southwest, passing four more ponds—these being larger—before reaching a lakelet worthy of a lunch break or a refreshing swim. Ahead, the trail continues southwest for 250 yards, then makes a steep ¼-mile climb south to a crest junction with the Pacific Crest/Tahoe-Yosemite trail. This you can then take ¼ mile south down to a spur trail that drops 100 yards to the northwest shore of **Dicks Lake**. See Hike 11 for more details about this lake and **Fontanillis Lake**.

Our route, Hike 20, takes the more popular tread, the one to Middle Velma Lake. We leave the junction by the ankle-deep pond as we climb northwest 50 yards to a slightly larger pond atop a broad saddle, and then descend a convoluted ¾ mile more or less in the same direction to a shallow, unnamed Velma lake. Don't camp at tempting shoreline sites, but rather farther back. When you reach its wide outlet creek, you may have to walk just upstream

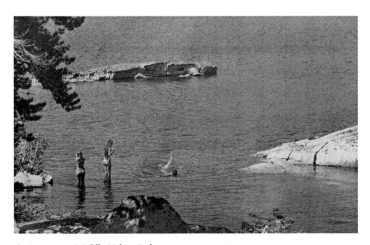

Swimmers at Middle Velma Lake

to find a dry crossing. If you were to go downstream 0.4 mile cross-country, preferably along the creek's northwest bank, you would reach Lower Velma Lake. This receives a lot less use than its trailside sisters and, being bedrock-lined, it has fewer mosquitoes. From the outlet creek our Velma Lakes Trail climbs 100 yards to a junction. By hiking south ⅓ mile on a trail from here, you can reach the north end of **Upper Velma Lake**. It is unique in having a grassy, semistagnant pond nestled on its bedrock island.

Only 180 yards past the Upper Velma trail junction, our westbound trail meets the Pacific Crest/Tahoe-Yosemite trail, which descends one mile from **Fontanillis Lake** and 2 miles from Dicks Lake to here. We take the PCT/TYT about 100 yards northwest, to where it curves west. Here you'll see **Middle Velma Lake**, and you can leave the trail for a quick descent to it. On weekends this lakeshore is crowded, for it has inviting water that tempts hikers to swim out to, dive from, or sunbathe on one or more of the lake's rock-slab islands. Rainbow trout also lure anglers to this sprawling lake.

Emerald Bay State Park
HIKE 21

Maps
4

Distances
0.8 mile to Emerald Bay, west shore
0.9 mile to Vikingsholm
1.2 miles to Eagle Falls
1.5 miles to Emerald Bay Boat Camp
2.0 miles to northwest corner of Emerald Bay
2.4 miles to Emerald Point
2.4 miles to Bonnie Bay

Directions to trailhead

From where Highway 50 leaves Highway 89 in South Lake Tahoe, drive 9 miles north on 89 to a large parking area on your right. This area is just ¼ mile past Eagle Falls Picnic Area's parking lot entrance. If you're coming from Tahoe City, drive 18½ miles south on 89. Lock your car, for thefts are all too common here. Be aware that the main parking lot and the picnic area's parking lot both can be completely full by 10 A.M. on a summer weekday, and earlier on weekends. Some desperate folks end up parking on Highway 89's shoulders as much as ¾ mile from the main parking lot. Be aware that the area you are about to enter is day-use only except for those staying in Emerald Bay's campgrounds.

Introduction

Lake Tahoe's beaches attract throngs of sunbathers, and the beach on the west shore of Emerald Bay is no exception. However, because it is the only Tahoe beach in this book's area that you have to hike to, it is less congested. Limited trailhead parking, which is usually full on summer weekends, also limits the number of Emerald Bay visitors. Most Lake Tahoe visitors would agree that this bay is the most scenic stretch of shoreline to be found along all of the mammoth lake.

Route description

The route is simple: follow a closed road down to Emerald Bay. By the start is a low knoll, which provides you with a commanding view of Emerald Bay as well as of the deep canyon to the southwest. Huge glaciers repeatedly descended this canyon, but barely eroded it, and in the bay, Fannette Island stands as testimony to glacial impotence. (When basal glacial ice meets an obstacle such as this, it melts, flows around it, and refreezes—not a process that erodes rocks.) The glaciers were at least as high as the moraines they left, and therefore may have been about 700 feet thick. This was enough to bury the low knoll under ice, but only thin, stagnant ice. Hence during the last glaciation, old, foot-deep solution pockets were not planed away, nor was the bedrock polished smooth.

Before making your 400-foot drop to Emerald Bay, be sure to leave your pets behind—and not in a vehicle where they might expire in the summer heat. The closed road drops ⅔ mile to another one, from which you descend 120 yards south to where a trail heads past a former gardener's cottage down to the nearby beach of

Emerald Bay. Swimmers will find the bay's water very cold until early August, when it climbs into the low 60s and stays there until mid-September, when the park generally closes. Perhaps the two weeks after Labor Day are best, for the crowds have diminished and Lake Tahoe typically has dropped a couple feet, creating a sandy beach not enjoyed by earlier visitors. After about 0.1 mile more on the road, you meet a trail that heads over to the **Vikingsholm** as well as to a pier at the nearby beach. The site is usually open daily for tours from about July 1 through Labor Day, and then on weekends until the park closes.

The road then goes past restrooms, on the right, and also curves over to the Vikingsholm. Just beyond the road's end, from the back of the Visitor Center, the short Eagle Falls Trail starts west. Very soon, cool, lush vegetation gives way to brush-covered slabs, moments before you reach **Eagle Falls**. The falls are roaring when Emerald Bay State Park opens in May, and they continue to do so well into July. About 200 yards up this short trail, another trail branches left to bridge nearby Eagle Creek, then continues 1.6 miles to end at the campfire center located between Lower and Upper Eagle Point Campgrounds. This trail is not meant for day-hikers; rather, it is a use trail that allows Emerald Bay campers to

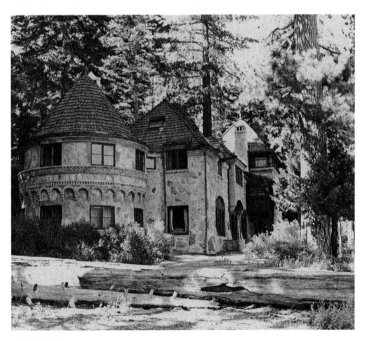

Vikingsholm

walk over to the Vikingsholm area. As it does not provide good access to the east shore of Emerald Bay, you will probably not find it worth the effort to explore.

The west shore is better, and it has ready access. From the Vikingsholm area or just north of it, take an obvious trail that traverses, usually just above the bay's west shore, for about ¼ mile to where it ends in the **Emerald Bay Boat Camp**, which is open to hikers who have made reservations. From the pier you take a road northeast 120 yards through the linear camp. Where the road turns left, away from the bay, your trail resumes. Ahead, the trail stays close to the shore, although thick brush limits access in most places. There is occasional shade, provided by white fir, Jeffrey pine, incense-cedar, and sugar pine. On a slope carpeted with bracken ferns the trail levels and you pass some of the tallest willows to be found in the Sierra Nevada. You'll recognize these 40-foot-high Scouler willows by their pale gray, aspen-like bark.

About 0.6 mile from the boat camp, the shore curves from northeast to east at the **northwest corner of Emerald Bay**, and you continue briefly northeast, starting to cross a low terminal moraine. Quickly you'll reach a trail branching east, which you follow for 0.4 mile out to **Emerald Point**. (Sometimes the start of this trail is obscure, although once on this popular route, its tread is obvious. Should you vault the low terminal moraine and start a descent, you've gone too far.) The mouth of Emerald Bay is extremely shallow, so much so that when Lake Tahoe lowers its level by 5 feet, one can boulder-hop halfway across the bay's mouth. Had the last glacier occupying Emerald Bay dropped just a bit more of its transported rockfall debris, the bay would have become "Emerald Lake," like similar Cascade and Fallen Leaf lakes south of it.

Emerald Point offers spectacular and instructive views. You can't miss a huge scar above the bay's end, which is the result of a December 26, 1955, rockslide caused by the construction of Highway 89 across a steep, fractured, unstable slope. Even these days, large blocks occasionally break loose to fall on the highway. Most of the land you see has been glaciated, and from your vantage spot you can study two enormous lateral moraines that flank the bay. These actually are thin glacial deposits that bury bedrock ridges; the amount of debris transported and then deposited by glaciers is much less than one would think. In the bay's distance you'll see Fannette Island, which you may have used in gauging your progress along your hike. Despite being repeatedly overrun by thick glaciers, the island still stands, since here, as elsewhere, glaciers performed very little erosion; however, these glaciers were thick enough to bury what is now your trailhead parking area under several hundred feet of glacial ice. Beside the parking area is a low knoll, popular with photographers, and on the up-canyon side of its gently sloping summit you'll find ancient, possibly pre-glacial potholes that have been unaffected by countless millennia of glaciation. One could argue that Emerald Bay's depth must be due to significant glacial erosion, but again, not so. About 2½ million years ago, before any glaciation and before Lake Tahoe, Emerald Bay was just the lower part of a canyon descending to the even lower floor of the Tahoe basin.

After your stay, return to the main trail or else make a 0.4-mile traverse across the low terminal moraine down to **Bonnie Bay**, where at times a boat or two may be anchored, and at times there may be up to a dozen or more swimmers, waders, sunbathers, and picnickers. To continue onward, see the next hike, which is described in the reverse direction south to this vicinity.

D. L. Bliss State Park

HIKE 22

Maps

2

Distances

0.1 mile to Rubicon Point

0.3 mile to the lighthouse

2.7 miles to Bonnie Bay

3.1 miles to northwest corner of Emerald Bay

3.5 miles to Emerald Point

Directions to trailhead

From where Highway 50 leaves Highway 89 in South Lake Tahoe, drive 11 miles north on 89 to the entrance to D. L.

Bliss State Park. If you're coming from Tahoe City, drive 16 miles south on 89. Take the park's road 2.4 miles down to its end. Halfway down this road, just 0.2 mile past the entrance station, is a small parking area, an alternate trailhead. From it one trail heads 100 yards east to the Rubicon Trail, while another one 60 yards north of it begins a crest route north to the road's end.

Introduction

Lester Beach is the prime attraction for the hundreds of campers who nightly crowd the park's five campgrounds. A few campers may visit "balancing rock" along the park's short nature trail, and even fewer hike the Rubicon Trail south to either Emerald Point or to Emerald Bay's Vikingsholm beach. Secluded shorelines await those who take this scenic trail. Pets are not allowed on this trail.

Route description

Just a few paces from the trailhead the Rubicon Trail reaches a junction. Branching right, a newer trail makes a switch-backing ascent 0.2 mile to a junction, from where you can traverse 70 yards southeast to the spur trail down to the lighthouse, mentioned below. Onward, the newer trail continues 0.8 mile, winding up and down a forested crest to a trailhead midway along the park's road. With poor views and sparse wildflowers, this trail is for those wanting exercise.

From the north end of this newer trail the Rubicon Trail makes a 150-yard, almost level traverse to the back side of **Rubicon Point**. From here you may see one or more use trails descending east to Tahoe's shore. One of them descends to the base of Rubicon Point, from where bathers can dive into the lake's chilly water. The water warms to the low 60s by mid-September, just when the state park is about to shut down.

We leave the back side of Rubicon Point, ascending shady, steepening slopes. Fortunately, a protective rail is present on the steeper slopes, for a slip there could be fatal. Just before the trail turns briefly west, you'll spy the old lighthouse, a small wooden structure resembling an outhouse, perched at the brink of a cliff about 60 feet above our trail. Where the trail bends west, you have dramatic views from atop a precipitous point just east of the trail. The east face of this point plus the nearby overhanging pinnacles together offer challenges for roped rock climbers. From its back side the point is a safe, easy climb, and you can gaze into Tahoe's deep, deep-blue depths. In 1970 you could see objects as much as 100 feet down, but by the mid-1990s you could see them only about 70 feet down. The clarity should not decrease much more, thanks to many stringent measures taken to restrict nutrient flow into the lake, which will reduce the algal growth rate.

Climbing briefly west, our route passes some trailside pinnacles and immediately meets a trail that climbs steeply to a small flat and a junction with a newer trail. From here a spur trail descends equally steeply to the **lighthouse**. At one time it must have commanded quite a view, but today tall conifers block it.

On the Rubicon Trail we now climb gently south, heading toward usually unseen Mt. Tallac, the most prominent peak above Tahoe's west shore. We see it, and most of Lake Tahoe, from a large trailside boulder found where the trail turns from south to southwest. Continuing on, we quickly reach two former roads about 25 yards apart. They unite in about 65 yards, then lead 35 yards to the park's road. From that alternative trailhead the lighthouse is ⅔ mile away, whereas it is only ⅓ mile from the Rubicon trailhead.

The Rubicon Trail now briefly climbs through a dense forest of white firs. These are so closely packed that they have shaded out huckleberry oaks, which once thrived when sunlight was more abundant. In this viewless forest we start a one-mile descent to Tahoe's shoreline. About ⅓ mile down it you may notice a former burn, on your right, where charred fir snags have been replaced with tobacco brush. Given time, these aromatic bushes will be overshadowed by firs.

A pair of switchbacks offer us a fine lake view, and they mark the approaching end of our descent. Just past them we meet the first of several use trails that descend to the bouldery shoreline. Here, 2 miles from the trailhead, you have your first easy access to Lake Tahoe since Rubicon Point. In the next ¼ mile you pass about a half-dozen access trails, then climb briefly to a springfed creeklet, the only lasting, trailside flow between our trailhead and Emerald Bay. A short, moderate climb takes us to a point with a great lake view, then we take short switchbacks down almost to the shoreline. Next we climb over a low rise to arrive at usually tranquil **Bonnie Bay**, a small half-moon, less than 100 yards across, along the shore of Lake Tahoe. Boats occasionally anchor in this photogenic bay, but in July and August, when the lake temperature rises into the low 60s, you're likely to see (fool)hardy swimmers (including the author), or at least waders. A fair number of large boulders lie just below the surface—a hazard for boaters but a boon for

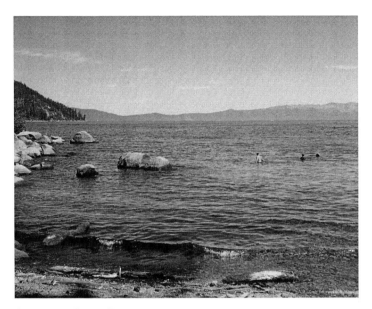

Swimmers in Bonnie Bay

swimmers, since you can make short, brisk swims from one submerged boulder to another, stand up on each to warm in the afternoon sun (sometimes appearing to be walking on water), and ultimately almost reach the open lake.

The previous hike describes the rest of the Rubicon Trail to and along the shore of Emerald Bay over to the Vikingsholm. If you've hiked this far, you'll probably want to visit Emerald Point, about 0.8 mile farther, although this spot is reached with less effort and distance from the previous hike. You first climb over a low terminal moraine left by the Emerald Bay glacier, and about 0.4 mile from Bonnie Bay reach a trail branching left, winding another 0.4 mile east to **Emerald Point** (if you miss the lateral trail, you'll momentarily arrive at the **northwest corner of Emerald Bay**.) The last part of the previous hike elaborates on Emerald Bay's glaciation. Glaciers did not carve out the bay, popular myth to the contrary.

Tahoe-Yosemite Trail to Middle Velma Lake

HIKE 23

Maps

2 and 3

Distances

4.6 miles to Lake Genevieve
4.9 miles to Crag Lake
5.7 miles to Hidden Lake
5.9 miles to Shadow Lake
6.3 miles to Stony Ridge Lake
8.1 miles to Rubicon Lake
9.1 miles to Phipps Pass
12.0 miles to Pacific Crest Trail
13.1 miles to Velma Lakes Trail
13.4 miles to Middle Velma Lake

Directions to trailhead

From where Highway 50 leaves Highway 89 in South Lake Tahoe, drive 3.2 miles northwest on Highway 89 to the Lake Tahoe Visitor Center. Get your wilderness permit here, then continue 13¼ miles on Highway 89 to a closed road just 230 yards past the Meeks Bay Campground entrance. If you're driving from Tahoe City, follow Highway 89 south 2.2 miles to the William Kent Visitor Center, get your wilderness permit, and then continue 8 miles to the trailhead, just 250 yards past Meeks Bay Resort. Park where you can find space anywhere along the highway. This trailhead usually has wilderness permits for *day users*.

Introduction

This relatively easy backpack route is along the subdued, northernmost part of the Tahoe-Yosemite Trail, which rewards you, starting 4½ miles in, with one lake right after another. Those who choose to take another trail down to Highway 89 should then be able to ride a T.A.R.T. bus back to the trailhead. First verify that these *seasonal* public buses are running between South Lake Tahoe and Tahoe City.

Route description

The Tahoe-Yosemite Trail starts west along a gated road and takes us through a forest of white fir, incense-cedar, and lodgepole, ponderosa, and sugar pines. After 1⅓ miles our road nears the upper end of a grassy swamp, on the left, and here a trail branches right. Ahead, the road ends in Vs mile at the site of former Camp Wasiu. On the trail we climb moderately for 0.4 mile up to a seeping trailside spring, and then continue up a gentler gradient to Meeks Creek. Its banks abound in wildflowers, thimbleberries, and bracken ferns as well as alders and willows.

Our ascent now becomes almost negligible as we progress southwest, enter Desolation Wilderness, and parallel the usually unseen creek along a large, mostly forested flat. We hike through the south edges of three dry meadows that sprout variable amounts of lupine and mule ears, and offer possible camping near their border. Beyond the last one we parallel the creek up a moderate ascent, then reach a second forested flat. Up here red fir, Jeffrey pine and western white pine have replaced their lower-elevation look-alikes: white fir, ponderosa pine, and sugar pine. Incense-cedar was the first to drop out, but a somewhat similar tree, the juniper, will be seen on exposed rocky benches above. Lodgepole pine—an inhabitant of several vegetational, climatic, and edaphic zones—remains with us.

We angle south gently down to a bridge across Meeks Creek, this locality having possible camping. Now we climb moderately up a path that arcs east into a shady, moist, red-fir-forested cove rich in vine maple, currant, thimbleberry, and fireweed. Then, winding southwest up the cove's south slope, we soon arrive at a much drier, more open ridge, a good resting spot from which we can just barely see Lake Tahoe. Now we climb southeast for a short, pleasant stretch beside cascading Meeks Creek as we hike up to shallow, relatively warm **Lake Genevieve**, lowest of the Tallant Lakes. In 1895, California's Fish Commission authorized the stocking of these lakes with Great Lakes Mackinaw fingerlings. When fully grown, these trout top 30 pounds. They migrated down Meeks Creek into Lake Tahoe, grew, and were eventually blamed by Tahoe anglers with destroying Tahoe's native cutthroat trout. Since all large trout cannibalize smaller trout, the Mackinaws weren't the only culprits. Besides, unrestricted commercial fishing had been going on for decades, first to feed the mining populations in western Nevada's silver mines, then later to supply more distant markets, and very little effort had been put into restocking the lake. (In like manner, the forests were mowed down to provide mining buildings, and then the razed slopes were abandoned.)

Along Lake Genevieve's northeast shore you may see the old, little-used Lake Genevieve Trail, which rambles 2⅔ miles over to the upper part of General Creek. There are campsites around this lake, some even with a good view of dominating 9054-foot Crag Peak, but since most of them are within 100 feet of the lake, you should move upstream and quickly reach larger, more appealing **Crag Lake**, beyond which Crag Peak rises in all its granite glory. Like Lake Genevieve downstream and Stony Ridge Lake upstream, Crag Lake has a low dam. Along its northeast shore are environmentally incorrect trailside campsites. Secluded, more appropriate sites exist along the lake's opposite shore.

Beyond Crag Lake your trail quickly guides you to a boulder-hop of Meeks Creek, and then you encounter a spur trail on a ridge just beyond it. This trail descends to shallow **Hidden Lake**, nestled near the foot of Crag Peak. Climbers wishing to climb moderately difficult Class 5 routes up its 400-foot northeast cliff should consult Carville's guide, mentioned under "Recommended Reading and Source Materials."

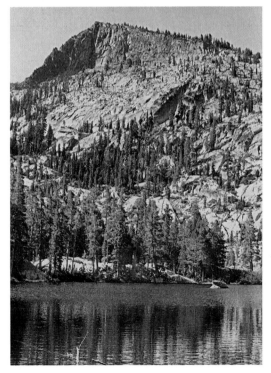

Crag Peak over Hidden Lake

From the Hidden Lake trail junction, we climb up the ridge, a lateral moraine, and then curve east to another ridge, this one being a recessional moraine. Behind it lies **Shadow Lake**. Given enough time, all lakes face extinction, and this lake is well on its way. Sediments have filled it to such an extent that water lilies have invaded its southern half. Close behind them in the marshy water are water-loving grasses and wildflowers. Pursuing them on mucky soil are currants and alders. In time the lower half may become a meadow, while the upper half may sprout lodgepole pines and mountain hemlocks. However, before this happens, a glacier—like dozens of previous ones—will advance down the Tallant Lakes canyon, obliterating sediments, soil, and vegetation.

Leaving this swampy lake behind, we hike up a moderately graded trail that momentarily becomes steeper as it climbs alongside Meeks Creek, whose water is tumbling in cascades and rapids down a granitic gorge. Above the gorge we reach **Stony Ridge Lake**, largest of the Tallant Lakes. Here, the best campsite of many available may be the one above its north end, just across a low dam. Our trail contours the long, southwest shoreline, briefly crosses some mafic rocks and fords several wildflower-bordered creeks. The dark, mafic bedrock is similar to granitic bedrock in that it was intruded from below up into overlying rocks that have since been eroded away. It differs in that it is much richer in iron and magnesium—hence the darker color.

At the lake's southwest corner we cross and immediately recross the lake's inlet creek, proceed south along the west edge of a boggy meadow, and then, near an impressive, low-angle cliff of granodiorite, start up a series of well-graded switchbacks, bounded by two tributaries. After almost reaching a steep, churning cascade we turn onto the last switchback, climb southwest, and get hemlock-framed views below of Stony Ridge Lake and its damp meadow. We soon curve south into a little willow-lined creek cove, bordered by steep vertical-jointed cliffs. Now a short climb southeast past a tiny tarn takes us to the west shore of **Rubicon Lake**. Dammed by a ridge of resistant bedrock, this lovely lake is the highest of the Tallant Lakes. Because they form a line of "beads" along the creek that connects them, they are called *paternoster* lakes, after their resemblance to beads on a rosary. Fairly close to the water is a good campsite under mountain hemlocks and lodgepole pines. The lake's water is nippy, reaching at best into the low 60s, but a tempting rock just off the west shore beckons one to jump into the invigorating, clear water. After you climb out to bask atop this rock, you can peer over its edge and watch trout swimming lazily below.

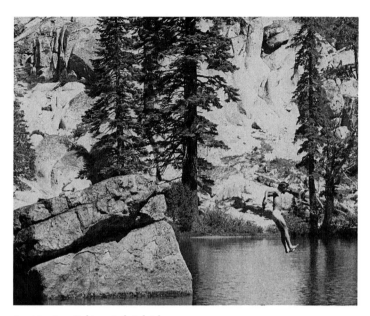

Jumping into Rubicon Lake's brisk waters

Above the lake's south end we reach an unmaintained trail that descends to the Grouse Lakes, which are a bit stagnant, and then 15 yards beyond the junction we top a saddle. The TYT then switchbacks up to a granodiorite outlier, just beyond which we can look back at it and see how joints really control its angular shape. We pass a small gully, snowbound as late as early August, then reach a switchback. Before climbing any farther, you might rest under a juniper or pine and enjoy the view in the southeast. Looking beyond the north end of Fallen Leaf Lake, we see Tahoe Mountain immediately above it, and from its slopes a long, level ridge—debris left by glaciers—extends southwest. Although this ridge, a glacial moraine, towers up to 900 feet above the lake, that doesn't mean these deposits are 900 feet thick. If we were to tunnel into them, we would find granitic bedrock beneath these *surficial* sediments.

A switchback leg north takes us higher up the joint-controlled rocks, and then our trail climbs moderately southward and crosses a gully just before skirting above **Phipps Pass**, the shallow saddle on your left. Just beyond the pass, the trail almost tops a crest on your right, and from it you could descend 320 feet down a steep slope to isolated camping near cold, circular Phipps Lake.

The route ahead, except for a few trivial gains, is all downhill. Our trail traverses granitic slabs and boulders along the southeast slope of Phipps Peak, named after General William Phipps, who settled along his ("the General's") creek near Sugar Pine Point. We encounter a spring, then swing around to the peak's open south slope, from which we can see the Velma Lakes in the gray, granitic basin below, and the rusty, metamorphic summit of Dicks Peak towering above it. The contact between the two rock types is clearly evident.

On the TYT we curve northwest, re-enter an open forest of mountain hemlocks and lodgepole, western white, and whitebark pines, perhaps pass some raucous Clark nutcrackers flying from tree to tree, and then come to within 30 yards of a ridge. Our route now descends southwest, then traces three long, well-graded switchback legs down to a junction with the Pacific Crest Trail. Along this descent we thrice cross a trickling creek and we pass many large red firs. Some of the older firs, now in the process of decay, have had their rotting trunks excavated by busy pine martens—larger cousins of the weasel—who chase down ground squirrels, which might also nest in these rotting trunks.

At the junction, we're only about a mile from and 200 feet above Middle Velma Lake, so we head down to this swimmer's paradise. The trail makes a moderate, generally viewless, descent to the lake's outlet creek, which all too often gets hikers' feet wet. The acres of soggy soil found in this forested flat prove to be a fantastic breeding ground for mosquitoes. Before August you'll want to scamper south along the trail trying to evade the pesky critters. After skirting past the southwest arm of Middle Velma Lake, you climb briefly to a junction with the **Velma Lakes Trail**. West, this trail descends to Camper Flat (described in Hike 11). East, this trail, also functioning as the PCT, TYT, and TRT, traverses 0.3 mile to a junction above the south shore of **Middle Velma Lake**, the arbitrary end of our hike. Just 70 yards before this junction, you have a good view of the lake and may want to descend to popular campsites near its shore. From the junction you can follow Hike 20 in reverse 4.4 miles out to the Eagle Falls trailhead along Highway 89 above Emerald Bay.

General Creek Trail

HIKE 24

Maps

2

Distances

3.5 miles to Lily Pond

5.3 miles to uppermost General Creek crossing

7.3 miles to Duck Lake

7.5 miles to Lost Lake

Directions to trailhead

From where Highway 50 leaves Highway 89 in South Lake Tahoe, drive 18¼ miles north on 89 to the entrance to General Creek Campground. Immediately past an entrance station (day-use fee required), branch left and head briefly east to the first parking lot on your left. Park in this eastern lot near its south edge.

Introduction

In Sugar Pine Point State Park, lower General Creek is flanked by two main trails, giving visitors many access points to the creek. Backpackers will find Lost Lake quite rewarding, for it is warm as Sierra lakes go. It even has a huge granite slab on which you can sunbathe. Leave your pets at home, since they are not allowed on the park's trail.

Route description

Take a paved bike path east along the south edge of the park's eastern parking lot, and in 60 yards reach a dirt trail branching south. On this trail you skirt along the perimeter of giant General Creek Campground, soon turn west, and then stay along the rim of a minor gorge cut by the creek. We pass campsites on our right and paths down to the creek on our left, then leave the rim for a quick junction with a closed road coming 0.1 mile from its start opposite campsite 150. If you happen to be camping at or near this site and begin your hike from it, then you can subtract 1.1 miles from all of the above distances.

Now on the one-lane closed road, we strike a level ¼ mile southwest to a junction with a second closed road, and are confronted with a choice of two equally long routes to upper General Creek, Duck Lake, and Lost Lake. The north-bank route is shadier and wetter, and before mid-August can have a mosquito problem. However, its vegetation is more diverse, and it is the shortest way to Lily Pond.

If you take the north-bank route, you'll hike ¾ mile along your closed road, passing midway along this stretch a glade with ferns and thimbleberries. Just before reaching General Creek, the road dies out in a lupine field, and a trail takes its place. This trail, becoming narrow, rocky, and quite winding, goes a shady mile southwest to a junction immediately past a gully. From it you can ascend a ⅓-mile trail to the south shore of **Lily Pond**, which for all but serious nature lovers is not worth the effort. The terrain is boggy and, through July, the mosquitoes are bad. This shallow pond nurtures yellow pond lilies, and it also supports a healthy crop of tall bulrushes. Like all of the park's species, these two plants are protected, although Indians formerly ate both. The bulrush in particular was highly desirable. One would eat the green shoots raw, or wait until autumn and make flour from the plant's roots. Its seeds, too, could be crushed and eaten. Furthermore, the stalks were useful for weaving bed mats and similar articles. From the junction with the Lily Pond trail, the north-bank route turns southeast and winds 100 yards to the south-bank route, the junction lying at the fringe of an aspen grove.

The south bank route, mostly a road, begins by first crossing General Creek. Use a nearby footbridge to keep your feet dry. Back on the road, you then quickly reach another road. Eastward, this goes 1 mile to Highway 89, opposite the state park's entrance to its Lake Tahoe shoreline day-use area (which has additional hiking opportunities). We go westward and parallel usually unseen General Creek upstream, passing granitic boulders dropped by a melting, retreating glacier. Soon we enter a long, thinly forested flat, which offers views of the two huge lateral moraines that border our creek valley. Their ridges are about 500 feet above us, and the glaciers that left them were at least 500 feet thick. The views disappear after about a mile of southwest hiking as we enter a thick, shady forest and soon bridge General Creek. Beyond it the road rapidly diminishes to a trail, reaching the aspen-grove junction about 0.4 mile beyond the creek. In early season this path can be quite soggy, and then you'll want to take the north-bank route.

From this junction we head south on a sometimes poor tread, which in ¼ mile improves as the trail turns westward, climbing to drier terrain. Jeffrey pines, lupines, and mule ears now line much of the trail, each species producing a pleasant, though often subtle, aroma. (Walk up to a large pine and stick your nose in a bark furrow. Smell like butterscotch? vanilla?) Beyond the state-park boundary, we're in for an easy 1¼-mile climb through National Forest lands, which offer the first camping possibilities. We then make our uppermost crossing of **General Creek** immediately below a lovely triangular pool and now, briefly on private land, climb a steep, rocky, ducked route to a closed jeep road. The road, which is just within National Forest land, winds 250 yards west to General Creek and thence back onto private land. We, however, start east, then immediately curve south, crossing the creek from Duck and Lost lakes in 0.8 mile, then recrossing it in an equal distance.

About 230 yards past your second creek crossing you'll come to an old logging spur left that drops 100 yards south to lodgepole-fringed **Duck Lake**, which is shallow enough to wade across. The main road curves right, climbing up to a second spur road, this one dropping north 200 yards to beautiful **Lost Lake**. Although past logging is evident along the main road to these two lakes, a swath of trees ringing each lake was spared the axe. You'll find a large campsite by Lost Lake's knobby south-shore peninsula and more-secluded ones along the path that circles this fine swimming lake.

Lovers Leap

HIKE 25

Maps
6 (and
optionally, 5)

Distances
1.2 miles to Lovers Leap

Directions to trailhead

See Hike 9's trailhead directions to Camp Sacramento. From its entrance, take the camp's road briefly east to a bridge over South Fork American River and immediately beyond the bridge you'll find trailhead parking for several vehicles on your left. The actual trailhead is 0.1 mile farther up the road, just past where it goes between two main buildings. Trail mileage is measured from the trail's start, since most of the hikers will be visitors staying at Camp Sacramento. This camp provides outdoor family vacations for Sacramento residents and, if space allows, for non-residents.

Introduction

This short ascent takes you up the easiest route to the summit called Lovers Leap. There are dozens of extremely difficult climbing routes up its nearly vertical northwest face. From the top you can see Pyramid Peak, the lateral moraines of Pyramid Creek, and much of the deep South Fork American River canyon. You may even see a climber or two, complete with high-tech climbing paraphernalia.

Route description

At the trailhead you can borrow a nature pamphlet that identifies common trailside plants, the numbers in the pamphlet keyed to numbered trailside posts. The trail immediately enters a ski-lift clearing, then re-enters forest cover and crosses several seasonal creeks. Along each creek you may see thimbleberry, lungwort (bluebell), tiger lily, corn lily, tall larkspur, red columbine, lupine, common monkey flower, and sunflowers such as arnica, senecio, and aster. Since each species has its own time for blooming, you may not see all these in bloom, but you may see others. Associated with the wildflowers are bracken fern, dogwood, alder, and aspen. Soon we spy the silvery plumes of Horsetail Falls in Pyramid Creek's canyon, north of us, and then encounter drier slopes on which thrive chinquapin, manzanita, snow bush (whitethorn), and huckleberry oak together with their wildflower associates.

The trail takes us just above a saddle that separates a low summit, on the right, from the main slope. Beyond it the climb steepens and switchbacks up to a junction on the weathered, gravelly ridge of **Lovers Leap**. Ahead, the Lovers Leap Trail descends over 1000 feet in 1½ miles to Road 11N19. We walk briefly north past a few Jeffrey pines and scrubby huckleberry oaks and manzanitas to the brink of Lovers Leap. Be very careful if you want to get a look down the nearly vertical face; the gruss, or granitic gravel, is slippery! Also be careful not to jar loose rocks that might hit climbers below.

The long, steep face of Lovers Leap, *unglaciated* (contrary to earlier views) and structurally resembling Half Dome in Yosemite, is considered as one of the best climbing areas in the Tahoe Sierra. Nearly vertical joints account for the steepness of the face. The low knoll north of and below you has lower-angle joints, so its slopes aren't as steep. What sets Lovers Leap climbing apart from most other Sierra climbing is the great numbers of horizontal dikes that have infused this rock. Long before any of its granodiorite was ever exposed to the earth's surface, this rock was intensely fractured, mostly along horizontal planes, and fingers of a molten mass, rising from below, were squeezed into these fractures, later to solidify as veins that geologists call *dikes*. Because they are rich in quartz and feldspar and are virtually devoid of any dark minerals—which are the first ones to weather—these dikes are more resistant than their relatively dark-mineral-rich host body is. Consequently, the dikes stand out from the faster-weathering granodiorite face, thereby providing climbers with convenient ledges to reach for and to stand on, making otherwise nearly impossible routes considerably easier. When you have had your share of views, and on weekends have seen a climber or two, return the way you came.

Sayles Canyon and Bryan Meadow
HIKE 26

Maps
7 (and
optionally, 6)

Distances
4.3 miles to Pacific Crest Trail (via Bryan Meadow)
5.0 miles to PCT (via Sayles Canyon)
10.2 miles for complete Sayles Canyon/Bryan
    Meadow semiloop trip

Directions to trailhead

First see Hike 8's directions up Highway 50 to the Pyramid Creek Trailhead. From there continue 1¼ miles to the obvious entrance to Camp Sacramento, then drive another 2.7 miles east up Highway 50 (or 3.1 miles west from Echo Summit) to Sierra at Tahoe Ski Resort. Drive 1.4 miles up its paved road to a junction with a graded road, branching right. Take this road 2.0 miles, traversing a ski area before reaching the trailhead at road's end.

Introduction

The Sayles Canyon and Bryan Meadow trails, which climb appreciably, do not take you to any lake nor up to any spectacular viewpoint. Hence they will appeal to only a select few, perhaps equestrians, who let their horses do the work, and botanists, who may hike only part way. For those seeking quietude, this may be a good hike.

Route description

From the upper end of a parking loop the Sayles Canyon Trail climbs initially through a shady forest. You then ascend a bouldery, rocky tread southeast to scrub-vegetated granodiorite slopes and, before curving east around a low glacial moraine, can glance back and see Pyramid Peak towering above barely visible Horsetail Falls. Curving east between the moraine and a creeklet alongside it, we quickly reach a junction with the Bryan Meadow Trail, 0.6 mile from the trailhead. We'll be returning down it. After crossing the creeklet, we soon come to an alder-lined Sayles

Canyon creek tributary that descends from Bryan Meadow. Rather than ford the shallow creek where the trail does, head just upstream to a boulderhop crossing. Here, under lodgepoles, you'll find a nice, flat campsite near the creek's north bank.

Beyond the ford our verdant pathway climbs southeast up the stepped canyon floor, at times almost touching Sayles Canyon creek. We pass some large boulders—up to 20 feet high—then traverse through a meadow largely overgrown with willows, alders, and corn lilies before we ford lushly vegetated Sayles Canyon creek. Then we tread a moderately graded stretch of trail 0.4 mile east up to the northwest corner of grassy Round Meadow. Near the meadow's north edge, the trail starts out along the south side of a clump of willows, heads east-southeast to a quick crossing of trout-inhabited upper Sayles Canyon creek, and then diagonals east-northeast toward some corn lilies. Beyond them it reaches slopes at the forest's edge, from which the trail upward is blazed and ducked. Mosquitoes, abundant through mid-August, make this damp meadow an undesirable camping area in early and mid-season.

On a trail that is bouldery at first, we ascend north moderately up past red firs and lodgepole pines, parallel a linear corn-lily meadow eastward, climb steeply north, and make a long, relatively gentle climb southeast before curving east up to a saddle. Here we encounter the **Pacific Crest Trail**, which also coincides for some distance with the Tahoe-Yosemite Trail. To follow this trail southward, see Hike 27.

Tracing the Pacific Crest Trail northward, we climb to a low summit, which has weathered boulders but no views, then we gradually descend through an open forest of mountain hemlock and lodgepole pine, cross a mucky slough that annually sprouts a magenta field of blazing shooting stars, and reach a trail junction at the upper east end of **Bryan Meadow**. Here the Pacific Crest Trail turns east.

An old trail once cut straight down Bryan Meadow, and today a use trail still goes 50 yards west down to a small, poor campsite amid a cluster of lodgepoles. Our Bryan Meadow Trail begins north, but quickly curves west to a gully, and then parallels the north edge of Bryan Meadow. In a number of spots we walk along the meadow's thick soils, rich in humus and clay. Both hold a lot of water. The clay likely is eroded from volcanic sediments on slopes northeast of and high above the meadow. The result is a richer profusion of plant species than would be found growing in nutrient-poor granitic soils.

Beyond the meadow our trail traverses a slope while paralleling Bryan Meadow's creek, below us. The trail here is drier, for the slope has a typical cover of *gruss*—the chunky, residual quartz and feldspar crystals that are left behind after most of the dark minerals of granitic bedrock decompose and erode away. We descend a ridgecrest, switchback down its more-forested north slope, ford several branches of a creek, and then curve westward as we descend to a fairly large, forested flat. At the west end the creek tumbles down a steeper slope while our trail switchbacks down a sloping meadow. It then goes left and descends via more switchbacks through more-open forest down to the Sayles Canyon Trail, on which we retrace our steps to the trailhead.

Echo Summit to Showers Lake

HIKE 27

Maps
6 and 7

Distances
1.0 mile to Benwood Meadow
3.9 miles to Bryan Meadow Trail
4.8 miles to Sayles Canyon Trail
6.4 miles to Trail 17E16
8.3 miles to Showers Lake

Directions to trailheads

Drive up Highway 50 nearly to Echo Summit. The Pacific Crest trailhead is near the start of Echo Summit Sno-Park's road, which begins ¼ mile west of Echo Summit. Just 100 yards along it is a left-side parking area for about 8-10 vehicles.

For an alternate trailhead, drive 200 yards east of signed Echo Summit, turn south on a narrow spur road and follow it ⅓ mile to its end, with parking for several vehicles.

Introduction

This route is a long way in to Showers Lake, and may appeal most to equestrians and botanists. The route's greatest users, however, may be neither, but rather long-distance hikers doing part or all of either the Pacific Crest Trail, the Tahoe Rim Trail, or the unofficial Tahoe-Yosemite Trail. From the heart of Desolation Wilderness south to the Carson Pass area, these two trails share the same tread.

Route description

From the trailhead parking area, you make a level walk south to a parking area for the Echo Summit Sno-Park. From its south end you briefly take a broad path south to the base of a ski slope, where the Pacific Crest Trail, unless snowbound (often into early or mid-July), starts a conspicuous climb southeast, diagonaling up some lower slopes. The trail soon turns south, climbs moderately but briefly, then makes a meandering traverse, passing a spring 0.2 mile before winding down to a junction just above the northeast edge of Benwood Meadow, where you'll meet an older trail coming from the alternate trailhead.

This trail, 0.3 mile shorter than the main route, begins at a small flat just west of a cluster of summer homes. It winds southward past large boulders of a lateral moraine, which were left as the glacier began diminishing and retreating, perhaps about 15,000 years ago. The moraine, which blankets a bedrock bench and canyon slopes, today stands about 1100 feet above the Upper Truckee River's canyon floor, but at the glacier's maximum, its ice surface would have been several hundred feet higher. Soon the trail descends past a lily-pad pond, to the west, and crosses its southeast-flowing outlet creek. The pond resembles so many others one sees in the glaciated High Sierra, but it is quite distinct in its mode of origin. Instead of forming behind a recessional moraine, as many have, this pond was dammed between two lateral moraines. The huge Upper Truckee canyon lateral moraine blocked the creek's drainage eastward and another lateral moraine extending east from the north edge of Benwood Meadow blocked its drainage southward, thereby ponding up the creek. On the low Benwood Meadow moraine you traverse southwest and, just after spying the meadow, join the Pacific Crest/Tahoe-Yosemite trail.

Benwood Meadow is a popular goal among botanists, for it is readily accessible, and it contains a diverse array of native species. The PCT fortunately avoids this fragile environment, cir-

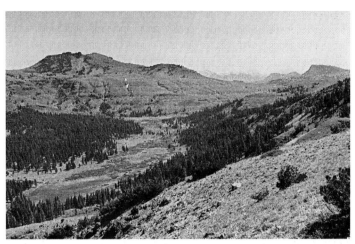

Red Lake Peak (left), Elephant's Back (far right) and the Upper Truckee River basin

cling around its west edge on somewhat drier, forested terrain. You then climb a brushy, rocky slope, cross a creek feeding the unseen meadow, and climb to a nearby switchback. Starting briefly west, you get your first view north at Lake Tahoe. Turning south, you climb ¼ mile to a shallow gap, having several more lake views along this moderate ascent. You next climb slopes up through an open forest, the terrain characterized by granitic outcrops and giant boulders.

About ½ mile past the gap you reach a crest saddle, which yields your route's best view, of the Upper Truckee River basin. Murky Round Lake, at the base of a volcanic palisade, is one of the most identifiable features. Just right of it and about a mile closer to you is Dardanelles Lake, which is nestled at the foot of a granitic cliff. Rising between the two lakes is flat-topped Red Lake Peak, which at 10,063 feet nudges out Stevens Peak by 4 feet to be the basin rim's highest point. Stevens is above and just left of Round Lake. Note how thick the volcanic deposits are in this area, roughly 2000 feet from Stevens Peak down to the Round Lake environs. These deposits, which are mostly andesitic, locally were episodically erupted from about 20 to 5 million years ago, and they eventually buried most of the Upper Truckee River basin. Over time, first streams and then glaciers removed most of the fairly erodible deposits from the basin, exposing its granodiorite landscape once again, little changed from what it had been at the time of burial.

Before moving on, note two more landmarks, both to the south-southeast. The first is the basin rim's low point, a saddle above the river's headwaters. Through this saddle the Pacific Crest Trail climbs south, heading for the Mexican border, about 1080 trail miles away. Just to the right of and beyond the saddle is Round Top, the glacier-gouged remains of an ancient volcano, which at 10,381 feet is the highest peak between Highways 88 and 4. Showers Lake, due south on a high, granitic bench, is unseen.

Beyond the viewpoint you skirt along the base of some intimidating granodiorite cliffs as you climb southeast. Just past them you reach the jump-across Benwood Meadow creek and above its westside can spy a small flat near the east bank. This is the site of "Six Pack Camp," in which you can pack six campers. Ahead, we climb rather steeply southwest to a lovely cove beneath a conspicuous dark cliff of volcanic rocks. Now we cross a sparkling creeklet that drains from the melting snowfield clinging to the upper slopes, then begin a reasonable ascent southeast to the gentle volcanic summit's forested east shoulder. Then we descend southwest on volcanic soils which, due to the porosity of their rocky particles here, are much drier. Flowers of mule ears and lupines, both with unmistakable scents, thrive in these soils. We get a brief view of peaks to the southeast but then submerge under the forest's cover once again as we descend, sometimes steeply, on granitic soils to a ravine with a tiny creeklet.

A short, easy climb west now takes us to a thickly cloaked saddle above Bryan Meadow, which has fair-to-poor campsites along its fringe. (You would do better to make a dry camp along our ridge.) Descending about 200 yards west to the meadow's east edge, we reach a junction from which the **Bryan Meadow Trail** (Hike 26) curves north. Should you need water, take this trail to the creek flowing from the lower end of the meadow.

Our Pacific Crest/Tahoe-Yosemite trail turns south, and after climbing 100 feet of elevation in that direction, we can see Pyramid Peak, the prominent summit of the granitic Crystal Range, on the northwest skyline. Through an open forest of mountain hemlock and lodgepole pine we now complete our easy climb to a low, viewless summit, then momentarily drop to a crest-saddle junction with the **Sayles Canyon Trail** (also Hike 26).

From the saddle your trail meanders along the broad crest for about ½ mile, then crosses a seasonally soggy, small meadow with a snowmelt creeklet. A rocky ascent of 300 feet gives way to a descent of 100 feet to a shallow crest gap. From it a faint use trail strikes east 250 yards down a linear meadow to a camp with a fine view, just beyond the meadow's far end. To the west, a similar tread descends 330 yards to the upper edge of a large meadow, then

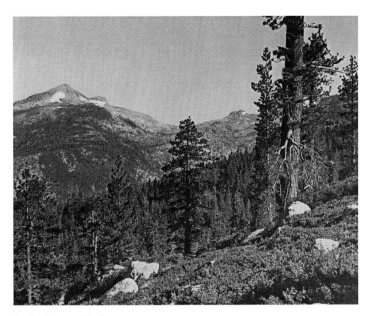

Sayles Canyon Trail

angles north-northwest for 130 yards to a camp among a cluster of lodgepoles. Both camps usually have water nearby through July. Climbing 0.2 mile from the gap, you'll next reach a near-crest junction with **Trail 17E16**. This eventually descends to Schneider's Cow Camp, and is described in Hike 32. Our route traverses southeast for ⅓ mile, then drops steeply, but briefly, south into a broad, glaciated basin. With volcanic flows and sediments above us and granitic bedrock below, we make an undulating traverse across the basin, always staying close to the contact between these two rock formations. While hiking this stretch, you might observe how each differs in kinds and abundance of plants, in soil production, and in the shape of the landscape. You may also note that volcanic-rock formations tend to have more streams and springs while granitic ones have the lakes. The first observation is true because many volcanic rocks are very porous, and can store water underground for year-round runoff, while granitic rocks are impervious, their water supply being stored in seasonal snowfields or briefly in shallow, gravelly soils. The second observation is true because the glaciers in this area were able to remove the loose volcanic sediments and carve basins in underlying, fractured granitic bedrock. Lakes then formed in these hollows when the glaciers receded. Volcanic rocks, being less resistant, are more easily planed smooth

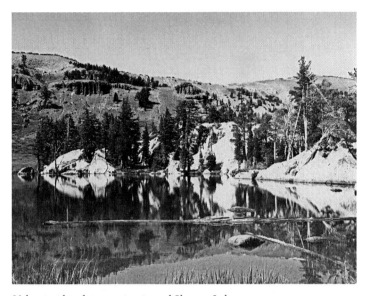

Volcanic ridge above granite-rimmed Showers Lake

or removed by glaciers, and hence hollows (and therefore lakes) rarely develop.

Our glaciated basin traverse takes us just beneath a precarious, overhanging volcanic point, beyond which we descend to where a use trail skirts southeast across willowy slopes that lie south of Showers Lake. For horses, this shortcut route is okay, but for hikers, the mire of mud negates the time saved. The official trail heads northeast through a gap in a linear wall of granodiorite that hides **Showers Lake**—a stone's throw—from us. Due to the obtrusive bedrock, the trail drops steeply down the lake's outlet creek, only to climb equally steeply up its other side to the lakeshore. However, in late season, you *might* be able to avoid this effort by fording, rock-hopping, or log-crossing the creek by the lake's outlet. Once across, you reach lakeside campsites shaded by mountain hemlocks, western white pines, and lodgepole pines. If you camp here before early August, be prepared for abundant mosquitoes.

Hawley Grade Trail

HIKE 28

Maps
6

Distances
1.9 miles to Highway 50

Directions to trailhead

From where Highway 89 branches south from southwest-climbing Highway 50, drive southwest ⅓ mile on 50 to South Upper Truckee Road, found immediately before a KOA Campground. Drive 3.7 miles south up this gently climbing road to where it curves left, you branch right on Road 1110 (hopefully signed for the Hawley Grade National Recreation Trail), and take this ¼-mile spur road past Bridge Tract homes almost to its boulder-blocked end, finding parking space for two or three vehicles about 50 yards before the end.

Introduction

Along the Hawley Grade you relive a bit of California's history by ascending the first wagon road to be built across the central Sierra. Hawley's Grade was a short-lived but key link in a trans-Sierra route to Hangtown and Sacramento. By 1850 Hangtown—today's Placerville—had become the unofficial capital of northern California's gold-mining region, and two years later a route of sorts was built from it to Johnson Pass—¼ mile north of today's Echo Summit—from where it dropped into Lake Valley. Drop it did, so steeply in fact that block and tackle had to be used to haul westbound wagons up it. An alternative grade had to be found.

A route over Luther Pass, to the southeast, was surveyed in the winter of 1854 for the purpose of providing a wagon road to Sacramento and Hangtown that would be better than Johnson Pass and also shorter and easier than the primitive Carson Pass route. That spring, Asa Hawley established a trading post in upper Lake Valley near a part of the Upper Truckee canyon's wall that quickly became known as Hawley's Hill. Construction soon began on a grade that would be gentle enough to safely accommodate wagons. Financed by private interests, this route—Hawley's

Grade—was completed in 1857, making it the first conventional wagon road to cross the central Sierra. Combined with a recently constructed Luther Pass segment, this grade fast became *the* route to take. In 1858 El Dorado and Sacramento counties improved western segments of this largely-one-lane toll road, making it far superior to the higher, longer-snowbound Carson Pass route to the south.

Timing couldn't have been better, for in 1859 silver was discovered in the Comstock Lode at Virginia Town, today's Virginia City. Traffic was reversed on this road as a flood of miners from California's gold fields scrambled east over this toll road to try their luck at or near Virginia Town. Alas, even as Hawley's Grade was constructed to channel westbound miners and pioneers into California's Mother Lode country faster than was possible along the Carson Grade, so too were plans made to convey miners and others east to the Comstock by a faster route. By the summer of 1860, a wagon-and-stage toll road—abandoned today—had been constructed down Meyer's Grade, then east to climb over Daggett Pass, situated above Tahoe's southeast shore. Hawley's Grade, briefly a shortcut that siphoned traffic from the Carson Pass route, now became the longer, unprofitable toll road.

Route description

From the boulders that today block the road, we start our hike up this historic grade by walking south about 100 yards, to where the road bends sharply and commences its climb to Echo Summit. From this bend, if you choose, you can first follow a trail 50 yards south to the tumbling waters of the Upper Truckee River. The road quickly reduces to a trail and we soon encounter a tangle of alders, bushes and wildflowers that take advantage of the pre-ponderance of springs and creeklets in this area. Beyond them we're on a narrow road again with more spacious vegetation. Scattered Jeffrey pine and other conifers break the monotony of the slope's mantle of huckleberry oak, and in shady spots bracken fern, thimbleberry, and spreading dogbane ("Indian hemp") add variety. In October the leaves of this diminutive hemp turn a bright yellow, making the plant one of the more conspicuous species. After the first fall frost, Indians would collect its stems in order to make string, which would be used for basket weaving and for bowstrings.

Midway along the ascent we reach our first good view north, then enter a gully down which a creek from Benwood Meadow and a pond north of it falls and cascades, splashing on the large boulders we must cross. Although our path across this gully is partly washed out, we have little difficulty crossing, and from its north side we can look back and see the tall volcanic cliffs that loom above Round Lake (Hike 30). Soon we get a glimpse of Lake Tahoe and spy trucks struggling up Highway 50's present Meyer's Grade. We can also see how growth along Tahoe's south shore has spread southward, transforming the forested valley below us into a suburb of South Lake Tahoe.

Our views of Lake Tahoe improve as we climb steadily north, but soon we veer west into a forest of white fir and Jeffrey pine and lose the views. Replacing them are the undesirable noise from traffic on Highway 50, which we're rapidly approaching, and the highly desirable aroma of a spread of tobacco brush. You can follow Hawley's Grade all the way to Highway 50's embankment, but this shoulderless highway is dangerous to walk along. When you see this embankment you can instead climb west up a shady gully and reach **Highway 50** at its junction with a narrow road leading south to the start of the Benwood Trail, Hike 27's alternate start. Most hikers, however, will retrace their route back to its trailhead.

Meiss Meadow Trail to Dardanelles Lake
HIKE 29

Maps
7

Distances
3.5 miles to Round Lake
4.0 miles to Dardanelles Lake

Directions to trailhead

See Hike 28's directions to a bridge over Upper Truckee River. Drive across the bridge and immediately turn right on Road 1111. Take this spur road ¼ mile, passing Bridge Tract homes before you come to a trailhead, which has parking for two vehicles, about 35 yards before a gate across the road.

Introduction

Since Hike 30 gets you to Round Lake and Dardanelles Lake in less distance and in less elevation gain, many hikers will skip Hike 29, particularly since trailhead parking is very limited, and there may not be any on summer weekends. Though longer and starting lower, this hike up the lower half of the Meiss Meadow Trail does have favorable attributes. It is much less used, and therefore more peaceful, it usually stays within earshot of a spring-fed stream, and wildflowers are more abundant.

Route description

This trail starts in a shady forest whose floor and slopes are adorned with a variety of colorful wildflowers. The trail starts to climb immediately from the left side of the road, and quickly reaches large boulders of a talus slope, which it traverses, and then it climbs steeply through the forest up to a more open, minor ridge. Here we contour toward a trickling creek, and make a steep ascent alongside it, then cross it just before topping a not-too-evident second minor ridge. Ahead is a third rise, but it is shorter and less steep than the first two, and the trail eases off and approaches a tributary of the Upper Truckee River. We make a relaxing stroll upstream beside this alder- and willow-lined creek, but then must climb moderately again as we reach a section of rapids. Eventually our ascent comes to a junction in a predominantly red-fir stand of conifers that also includes Jeffrey, western white, and lodgepole pines. The main trail continues south-southeast 0.2 mile gently up to a second junction at the more popular Big Meadow Trail (Hike 30), which climbs south mile to **Round Lake**.

If Dardanelles Lake is your goal, veer southwest from the first junction and ascend 30 steep yards toward the creek you've been paralleling—but first note the strange, 10-foot-high boulder you've seen downstream. This boulder broke off from the impressive volcanic palisade that towers above Round Lake. The cluster of smaller volcanic rocks that make up the large boulder you see are just a biopsy of one of the large volcanic mudflows one would see on Hike 30, which elaborates about the preponderance of these flows.

The spring-fed creek receives its water from subterranean channels that flow through the volcanic rocks downstream from Round Lake, ⅔ mile south of us. Across the creek the trail makes a traverse across a broad, low slope, first passing a second Round Lake creek, larger than the first, and then a lily-pad pond. After a quick descent, the trail reaches a third Round Lake creek, the one that leaves a dam at the lake's northwest corner and tumbles down a narrow, curving canyon. At one point these outlet creeks are almost a mile apart, before they finally merge only 200 yards upstream from our trailhead.

Our creekside journey downstream soon takes us past an aged patriarch—a seven-foot-diameter juniper—then past many creekside willow thickets to a ford of this creek. We tread across some low, glacially polished granodiorite slabs, and then climb southward on a ducked trail up a straight, easy, joint-controlled gully leading to rock slabs above the east shore of **Dardanelles Lake**. From its south shore rise the steep granodiorite cliffs of summit 8402, which, for climbers, are the reward of this long ascent. Nonclimbers will have to admit that the cliffs do add to the beauty of this shallow lake, which in midsummer warms to 70 degrees or more, making it ideal for swimming. Anglers can try to catch a

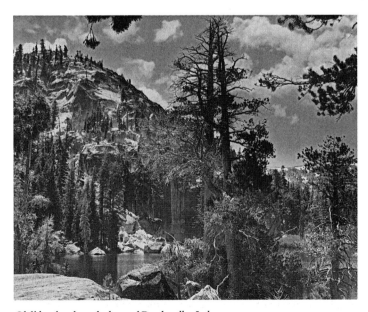

Cliff-bordered south shore of Dardanelles Lake

tasty brook-trout dinner. Late in the summer the lake's water becomes slightly cloudy, making it less attractive. Fair-to-good campsites exist among scattered junipers and lodgepoles on slabs bordering the east and northwest shores.

Big Meadow Trail to Round Lake
HIKE 30

Maps	Distances
7	0.8 mile to Big Meadow
	3.0 miles to Round Lake
	3.9 miles to Dardanelles Lake
	4.5 miles to Meiss Lake (via west route)
	4.8 miles to Meiss Lake (via Meiss Meadow Trail)

Directions to trailhead

From Echo Summit, Highway 50 drops into the Lake Tahoe Basin, reaching a junction with Highway 89 in 4.0 miles. Drive about 4½ miles south up this highway to the start of a long curve left, then another ¾ mile along it to where it straightens out and you turn left onto a paved road. (If you are driving northbound on Highway 89, this junction is about 3.3 miles west of Luther Pass.) This road quickly reaches the signed Tahoe Rim Trail's Big Meadow Trailhead facility. The Big Meadow Trail begins from the bottom parking loop.

Introduction

Because it has volcanic and granitic soils in various stages of development, the Upper Truckee River's uppermost basin supports approximately 300 species of wildflowers, shrubs, and trees, and it supports a similarly diverse invertebrate fauna. The Big

Meadow Trail is the most popular trail into this lake-dotted, volcanic-rimmed basin, which offers climbers some interesting routes. Most hikers go to Round Lake, the basin's largest lake, which strong backpackers can reach in about an hour.

Route description

From the bottom parking loop the Big Meadow Trail, doubling as the Tahoe Rim Trail, goes 240 yards to Highway 89, which you cross. Now you make a relatively short, moderate ascent via switchbacks completed by TRT volunteers in 2002. The upside is that you no longer huff and puff, as one did on the formerly steep ascent. The downside is that the route is now more inviting for mountain bikers, who can legally use this trail (and most other trails other than the Pacific Crest Trail and all trails in wildernesses). After the moderate, forested, bouldery ascent, the trail eases off to reach a junction, from which a trail, branching left, traverses 2½ miles east to Scotts Lake. Just 100 yards past the junction you reach the north fringe of well-named **Big Meadow**, and your trail quickly bridges trout-inhabited Big Meadow Creek. Throughout the 20th century, all of the Upper Truckee River drainage was cattle-grazing country, but now cattle are totally banned, making the trails, meadows, and lakes more attractive and wilderness-like.

Beyond the creek crossing, our path turns south again and we make a very flat traverse before we enter forest cover again, in a cluster of mature lodgepoles that trespass into the southeast corner of the meadow. Now our path winds south up a lodgepole-covered slope, which also is cloaked with clusters of red fir in some places and with open patches of mule ears and sagebrush in others. Near the top of your climb the grade eases and at just over 2 miles from the trailhead, you cross a broad, forested saddle.

On the fairly steep slope of volcanic rubble that we descend, the trees aren't as densely packed as were those along our ascent, so we can survey the basin we are entering. At the base of a prominent granodiorite cliff one mile west lies shallow, unseen Dardanelles Lake; above and beyond both stands a volcanic ridge, usually laced with snow and composed of many flows that are discernible by the naked eye. At the base of the massive volcanic cliffs ahead of us lies our unseen destination, Round Lake.

After passing some fine specimens of Jeffrey pine, whose deeply furrowed bark emits a butterscotch odor that permeates the warm air, we meet the Meiss Meadow Trail, which has climbed up a tributary of the Upper Truckee River. A gentle 0.2-mile descent along its aspen-covered banks will take you to a junction from where a 1.3-mile-long trail branches west to **Dardanelles Lake** (see Hike 29). We continue south, climbing up, down, and around on hummocky terrain of volcanic mudflow deposits and blocks. Our trail, now over fine-grained volcanic soils, is considerably dustier than the coarser-grained granitic soils we started on. Several minutes before we reach a flat above Round Lake's northeast shore, we pass one large large lava block that has a five-foot-long granitic boulder exposed in it.

Arriving at the northeast shore of **Round Lake**, we see it is different from all the other lakes of this guidebook's hikes. Bordered by volcanic deposits along its north, east, and south shores, the lake is brownish-green in color due to super-fine volcanic particles held in suspension. Since you'll probably not want to drink this water, hike 170 yards along the lodgepole- and cottonwood-lined east shore and obtain water from a trickling creek. Fair campsites are scattered about the northern half of the lake, the southern half generally being too vegetated and swampy. Perhaps the best sites are near the lake's outlet, where you'll find an old, 6-foot-high check dam. Apparently it is no longer in service, for the water level often is at the base of the dam, exposing a bathtub ring around the lake. From the northeast corner, follow a narrow path west past Jeffrey pines, junipers, sagebrush, mule ears, and buckwheat to a small campsite on a granodiorite bench just west of a head-high dam. Beneath red firs and lodgepoles you can take in superb sunsets that set the towering volcanic palisade east of you ablaze with color. Just east of this campsite is a small cove in which you can enjoy a refreshing swim. Fishing, however, is forbidden in the Alpine County part of this basin.

If you want to hike up to shallow, boulder-dotted Meiss Lake, you can reach it from Round Lake by two routes. The first is to start from the northwest campsites and follow a use path south along the west shore of Round Lake. At this lake's southwest corner you'll find more campsites, these shaded by lodgepoles growing on a flat bench above the lake. From this bench a faint use trail climbs south a short mile to **Meiss Lake**.

The second route to Meiss Lake is to hike south from Round Lake on the Meiss Meadow Trail. After one mile you reach a meadowy area with a conspicuous, entrenched creek. Leave the trail just before it crosses this creek and head cross-country ½ mile west to **Meiss Lake**. This second, slightly longer, route is preferable if you are carrying a heavy pack, for its terrain is easier than the first. Just 2.3 miles from Round Lake, the Meiss Meadow Trail joins

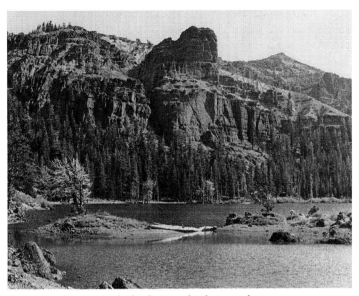

Towering volcanic palisades border Round Lake's east shore

the Pacific Crest/Tahoe-Yosemite trail in Meiss Meadow (see Hike 31). Meiss Lake is one of the warmest in the Tahoe area, for it is very shallow. Indeed, you can wade across it—too shallow for trout. If you use the lake's campsites—along its west shore—expect, until early August, plenty of mosquitoes.

Back near the creeklet dropping to Round Lake's northeast shore, the Meiss Meadow Trail passes an enormous block that, like so many others there, has broken off from the vertical-to-overhanging cliffs above. Climbers who like to go bouldering will find this an ideal block to climb. Since some routes are overhanging and others are as long as 40 feet, and since the holds aren't always secure, a top rope is desirable. More daring climbers may want to try the potentially dangerous deep fissures on the vertical cliffs above.

These mudflow cliffs are part of the Mehrten formation, which is an assortment of andesitic flows and deposits that here are up to about 2000 feet thick. From 26 to 5 million years ago thick andesitic lava flows sporadically poured from various Sierran volcanoes that probably resembled those of today's Oregon Cascades, and they covered an area from Sonora Pass north to Lassen Park and beyond. The *autobrecciation* of flows—the self-fracturing of a flow's rocks by its own movements—was responsible for the overwhelming quantity of *lahars*, or volcanic mudflows, which characterize the Mehrten formation. A lahar flows when an accumulation of fragmental debris becomes saturated with water. The extensive autobrecciation of these andesite flows produced a very abundant supply of fragments—"food" enough to feed hundreds of lahars like the ones that compose the thousand-foot-thick wall above Round Lake. Streams and then glaciers have removed most of the lahar deposits that once filled the southern part of the Upper Truckee River basin.

On Map 7, the Four Lakes look appealingly close and relatively easy to reach from Round Lake, Meiss Lake, or the Pacific Crest Trail. Basically, this is true, but there are a number of small ridges lying between the map's contours, and if you are not good at cross-country navigation, you can easily miss them. Only the relatively large, linear, southern lake is worth visiting, and folks have camped at it (try the granite bench above the east shore). All lakes are in prime mosquito lands, something to consider before mid-August.

Carson Pass to Showers Lake

HIKE 31

Maps
7

Distances
4.0 miles to Meiss Lake
5.0 miles to Round Lake
5.1 miles to Showers Lake

Directions to trailhead

Drive up Highway 88 to a curve with a parking lot, just ¼ mile west of the parking lot at Carson Pass. This pass is about 100 miles from Highway 99 in Stockton and about 20 miles from Highway 50 in the Lake Tahoe Basin.

Introduction

This walk along the Pacific Crest/Tahoe-Yosemite trail presents the hiker with a very scenic route to Showers Lake, the highest lake in the Upper Truckee River basin. The lake is a worthy goal in itself, but even if it were not, the hike to it across a glaciated volcanic landscape would justify the effort. The country traversed along this hike is among the Sierra's best for subalpine botanizing. Side trips include visits to Meiss and Round lakes.

Route description

From the trailhead at the northwest corner of the parking lot, first climb southwest and then round a ridge to make an undulating traverse northwest past junipers and occasional aspens to a gullied bowl. Both tree species release subtle scents, though these usually go unnoticed by the hurried hiker; they are often masked by the stronger scents produced by mule ears and sagebrush. After winding in and out of several gullies, you follow short switchbacks north, then traverse west to a junction with the Meiss Meadow Trail. Starting opposite a Woods Lake road junction 0.9 mile west of Carson Pass, this old trail climbs steeply to this junction in 0.5 mile, versus 1.3 miles for the scenic, leisurely PCT/TYT. In 110 yards your north-climbing trail tops a drainage divide at a saddle. Here you have a fine view to the south, dominated by 10,381-foot Round Top and flanked on the east by 9603-foot Elephants Back. Former glaciers grew outward from Round Top, and a giant one

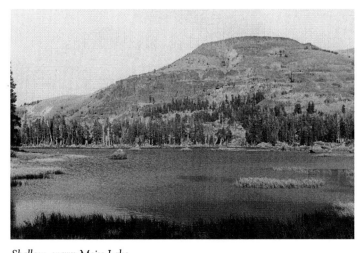

Shallow, warm Meiss Lake

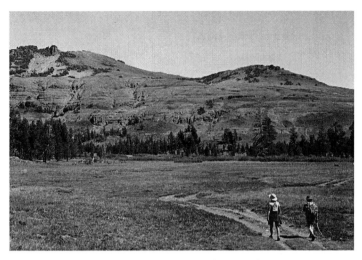

Stevens Peak (left) rises above the Upper Truckee River basin

advanced over our drainage divide and eroded a hollow in our saddle, which then filled to become today's shallow pond.

With most of the climbing behind us, we now make an
easy traverse ⅓ mile north along former jeep tracks to a junction,
where we angle left and descend tracks to a campsite by a jump-
across ford of the infant Upper Truckee River. We now have an
easy descent northwest, then pass through a gate, recross the river,
pass through a second gate and in a moment reach a fork. From
here, near cabins in giant Meiss Meadow, the Meiss Meadow Trail
heads 2.3 miles to the northeast corner of large, slightly cloudy
Round Lake (see Hike 30). You can follow this trail over a low,
broad ridge, reaching a lodgepole-fringed meadow in 0.5 mile.
From it you can then leave the trail and head cross-country 0.6
mile northwest down gentle slopes to the southeast shore of shallow, warm **Meiss Lake**.

Our main trail continues northwest, passing another tread
in ¼ mile, this one going to the meadow south of Meiss Lake. Just
before we meet our third river ford, we see the lake, and immediately before the ford a use trail provides the hiker with an easy ½-
mile meadow traverse to Meiss Lake. The meadow, sometimes dotted with cattle, is often damp if not downright boggy, particularly
near the south end of the lake, and until early August this wet
environment nurses a multitude of mosquitoes. Before mid-August
take the cross-country route to Meiss Lake. From mid-August

through mid-September this chest-deep lake is ideal for swimming or just plain relaxing.

After jumping across the Upper Truckee River for the last time (fishing prohibited), we head northwest along a meadow's edge and, just before crossing a shallow gap, may see a faint trail, on our left, which comes 2.1 miles from Schneider's Cow Camp (Hike 32). Just beyond the gap we descend north to a pond, and resume our lodgepole-and-meadow traverse. Our route soon curves left for an increasingly steep ascent to a broad crest. As we start a descent from it, we meet a second trail from Schneider's Cow Camp, 2.0 miles distant (also Hike 32). After a brief descent we reach campsites along the east shore of granodiorite-bound **Showers Lake**. An old horse trail still traverses northwest across willowy slopes south of the lake, but the slopes are very muddy, and hikers should avoid it.

The actual PCT/TRT/TYT route descends one side of the lake's outlet creek, only to climb up the other side. However, when water is not flowing swiftly over the lake's outlet, one can save about 0.2 mile by crossing at or just below the outlet. On the northwest shore is granitic bedrock, used for sunbathing and at some spots for diving into this usually cold lake. Also near this shore and to the south there are additional campsites.

Schneider's Cow Camp to Showers and Meiss Lakes

HIKE 32

Maps

7

Distances

2.1 miles to Showers Lake

2.9 miles to Meiss Lake

5.7 miles to Showers Lake (via long route)

Directions to trailhead

From Highway 99 in Stockton drive about 97 miles northeast up Highway 88 to Caples Lake Resort, above the north shore of Caples Lake. Continue 0.9 mile past the resort to a paved road, on your left. (Westbound drivers: this road is 3.0 miles west of Carson Pass.) Take this road ¼ mile to the Caples Lake Maintenance Station, and immediately past it turn right and drive up a graded road. Before August it can be muddy in several places, mostly in the first half-mile stretch. After 1¼ dusty miles you pass waterless Schneider Camping Area, on a broad ridge to your left, then continue 0.4 to a gate and a road fork. Park here.

Introduction

The shortest trail to Showers and Meiss lakes starts from near Schneider's Cow Camp. Ironically, this trail hasn't gotten much use in the past. The trail to Showers Lake has a short section along which you obtain one of the most expansive views to be seen anywhere in the Tahoe area.

Route description

From the fork in the road past Schneider's Cow Camp, you can start two routes to Showers Lake. The longer route starts by going up the road you drove in on, which quickly becomes a jeep road. The shorter route, which will be described first, starts by the east side of the road fork. This trail climbs 230 yards east to a barbed-wire gate, then climbs at a gradually steepening pace through cow country. Lodgepole stands give way to open spaces, which seasonally abound with many species of wildflowers. You leave most of the cows behind as you switchback steeply up to a crest saddle, passing a few whitebark pines before reaching it. Only 1.1 miles from the trailhead, this view-packed saddle is a worthy goal in itself. And for even better views you can go east cross-country along the crest, either ¼ mile northwest to peak 9325 or, preferably, ¼ mile southeast to peak 9422. From the saddle you see Meiss and Round lakes to the northeast, and above them see the volcanic palisades of the Upper Truckee River basin. To the left of these cliffs stands a distant granitic massif with 10,881-foot Freel Peak, the highest peak of the Tahoe Basin rim. The view to the southwest includes volcanic palisades above Kirkwood Creek, but Caples Lake and Round Top remain hidden.

From the saddle you gently climb a brief 85 yards to a junction. From it a trail drops 0.9 mile east down Dixon Canyon

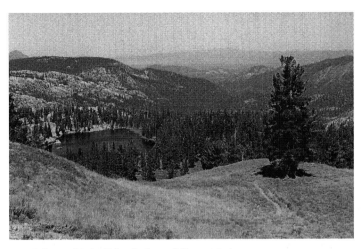

Mt. Tallac and Lake Tahoe lie beyond Showers Lake

to the Pacific Crest Trail (which here also coincides with the Tahoe-Yosemite Trail route). It is generally easy to follow, but the last 200 yards to the PCT are vague, bearing 110°. If you take this short trail, you won't have any trouble finding the PCT, but study this locale so you can find your trail if you plan to return along it (you may want to follow the last part of Hike 31 to Showers Lake). On the PCT this "junction" is about 180 yards south of a pond and 360 yards northwest of an Upper Truckee River ford. From the east side of that ford you can follow an often wet use trail ½ mile north to **Meiss Lake** (see Hike 31).

From the junction just beyond the crest saddle, the left trail climbs briefly and then descends, usually at a moderate grade. Before Showers Lake comes into view, stop and admire the astounding views, which are among the best in the whole Tahoe area. You can see from 10,776-foot Mt. Rose, above the north shore of Lake Tahoe, southward to 11,398-foot White Mountain, about 4 miles north of Sonora Pass. This 70-mile panorama includes, northeast to southeast: granitic Freel Peak, relatively close Stevens and Red Lake peaks, the very distant Highland and Arnot peaks—all above 10,000 feet. Lower prominences rising above the end of Upper Truckee River canyon are Reynolds Peak, the Nipple, Peak 9381, and, on the far right, broad-topped Elephants Back. Your panoramic views continue to a cluster of mountain hemlocks, by which you have the first view of your goal. Showers Lake. Distant Mt. Tallac, in eastern Desolation Wilderness, appears just above this lake, and to its left are the two summits of Dicks and Jacks peaks, in the heart of that wilderness. The isolated peak west of them is Pyramid Peak, the sentinel lording it over the southwest border of the wilderness.

The short descent to Showers Lake is rubbly and excessively steep. It's bad enough when dry, but after a storm, or when snowpatch-dotted in early season, you'll really slip and slide down this trail segment. Then, it's better to take the longer, alternate route. The steep descent moderates just before you reach the PCT, along which you have only a couple minutes' walk to campsites along the east shore of subalpine **Showers Lake**. If you camp here before early August, be prepared for abundant mosquitoes. This lake is one of the cooler lakes to be found in the Tahoe area, and most people will find swimming in it acceptable only in August, a couple of weeks after nearby snow patches have melted.

If you have a heavy pack or are on horseback, you may not want to make the steep descent to Showers Lake. For variety, hikers might plan to take the longer route to the lake, and then, with lighter packs, climb out via the shorter route just described. From Schneider's Cow Camp the longer route starts northwest up a jeep road, quickly passes a gate, and almost ½ mile from the start crosses a seasonal creek. About 40 yards past it you come to a trail, which you ascend steeply north. The trail rapidly swings left, and on an easier grade you climb west with views south to Caples Lake and Round Top Mountain.

About one mile from this hike's start the trail bends north, enters forest shade, and climbs to a nearby early-season creeklet. You cross it, parallel it upstream, climb to a subordinate crest, and then drop to a small flat. Staying close to the contact between volcanic rocks above and granitic ones below, you traverse north-northwest for ½ mile, passing two closely spaced springs midway to a trail fork. From here an old trail goes left, descending ¼ mile to die out on a broad ridge. Our trail briefly climbs north, then traverses east below the slopes of Little Round Top. Along this traverse you'll get a couple of views of Pyramid, Jacks, and Dicks peaks. From a reliable creek the trail angles north and contours 0.4 mile to an enormous trailside mountain hemlock, on your left—among the largest you'll find anywhere. About 90 yards past it you enter lands of the *Fallen Leaf Lake* 15-minute quadrangle and momentarily receive additional views of the three Desolation Wilderness peaks seen earlier. Our Trail 17E16 then curves east, drops to a spring-fed creeklet, and reaches the PCT in 200 yards. From here you follow the last part of Hike 27 south 1.9 miles to campsites along the east shore of **Showers Lake**.

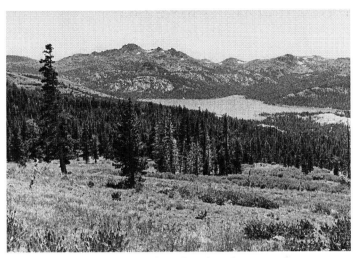

Round Top dominates the skyline beyond Caples Lake

If you're not ready to join the weekend crowd at Showers Lake, then descend about 300 yards north on the PCT to a saddle. From it a faint, discontinuous path strikes east 250 yards down a linear meadow to a camp with a fine view, just beyond the meadow's far end. To the west, a similar tread descends 330 yards to the upper end of a large meadow, then angles at 330° for 130 yards to a cow camp among a cluster of lodgepoles. Both camps are seldom visited, at least by humans.

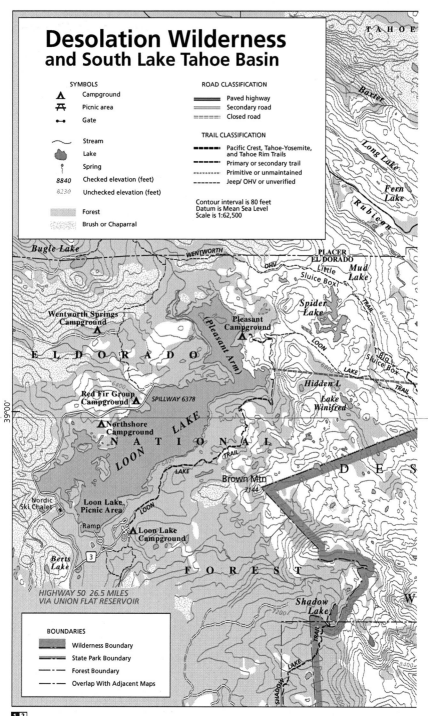

Desolation Wilderness
and South Lake Tahoe Basin

SYMBOLS

△ Campground

⊼ Picnic area

•⊶ Gate

〜 Stream

Lake

⌇ Spring

8840 Checked elevation (feet)

8230 Unchecked elevation (feet)

Forest

Brush or Chaparral

ROAD CLASSIFICATION

Paved highway

Secondary road

Closed road

TRAIL CLASSIFICATION

Pacific Crest, Tahoe-Yosemite, and Tahoe Rim Trails

Primary or secondary trail

Primitive or unmaintained

Jeep/ OHV or unverified

Contour interval is 80 feet
Datum is Mean Sea Level
Scale is 1:62,500

BOUNDARIES

Wilderness Boundary

State Park Boundary

Forest Boundary

Overlap With Adjacent Maps

Map labels: TAHOE, Baxter, Long Lake, Fern Lake, Rubicon, Bugle Lake, WENTWORTH, OHV, PLACER EL DORADO, Little Sluice Box, Mud Lake, Spider Lake, Wentworth Springs Campground, Pleasant Campground, (Pleasant Arm), LOON, Big Sluice Box, E L D O R A D O, Red Fir Group Campground, SPILLWAY 6378, LAKE, Hidden L, Lake Winifred, Northshore Campground, N A T I O N A L, LOON LAKE, TRAIL, D E S, Brown Mtn 7144, Nordic Ski Chalet, Loon Lake Picnic Area, LOON, Ramp, Loon Lake Campground, Berts Lake, 3, F O R E S T, HIGHWAY 50 26.5 MILES VIA UNION FLAT RESERVOIR, Shadow Lake, W, SHADOW LAKE

Map 1 – Loon Lake Area

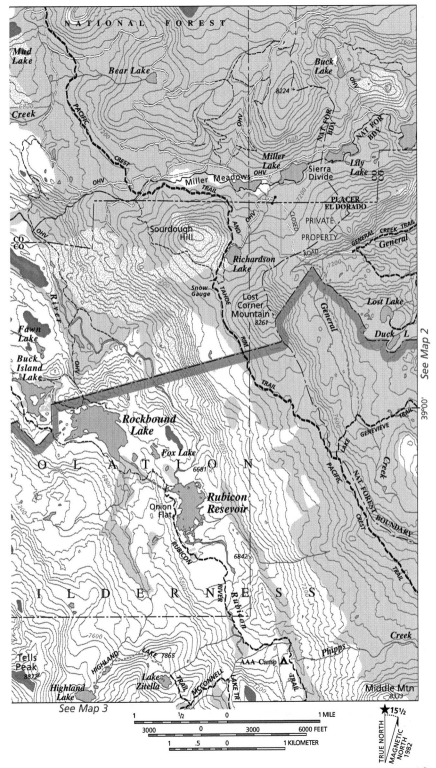

See Map 2

See Map 3

1   ½   0   1 MILE

3000   0   3000   6000 FEET

1   .5   0   1 KILOMETER

★15½

TRUE NORTH
MAGNETIC NORTH 1982

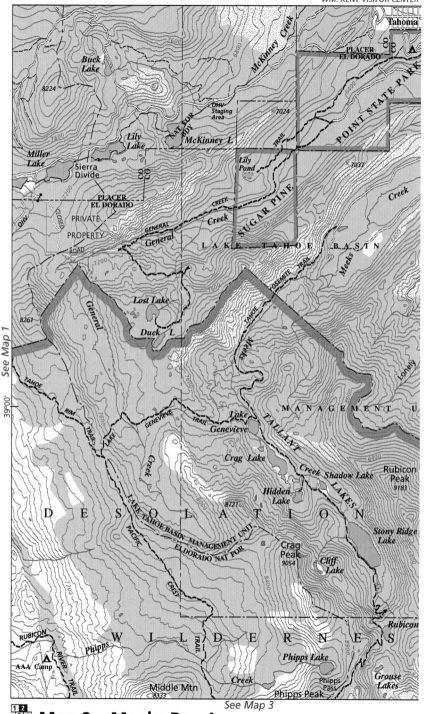

Map 2 – Meeks Bay Area

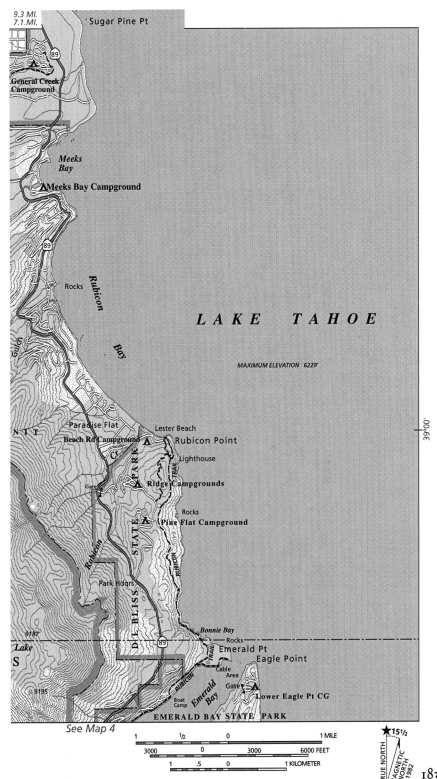

9.3 MI.
7.1 MI.

Sugar Pine Pt

89

General Creek
Campground

*Meeks
Bay*

▲Meeks Bay Campground

89

Rocks

Rubicon

Bay

Gulch

L A K E   T A H O E

MAXIMUM ELEVATION 6229'

39°00'

N T T   Paradise Flat   Lester Beach

Beach Rd Campground   ▲ Rubicon Point

Lighthouse

Gate   ▲ Ridge Campgrounds

RUBICON TRAIL

Rocks

▲ Pine Flat Campground

Rubicon   RUBICON

STATE   PARK

Park Hdqrs

9187

D L   B L I S S

Lake

S   89   Rocks   *Bonnie Bay*

TRAIL   Emerald Pt   Eagle Point

Cable
Area

9195   RUBICON TRAIL   Gate   ▲ Lower Eagle Pt CG

Boat
Camp   *Emerald   Bay*

EMERALD BAY STATE   PARK

See Map 4

1	1/2	0		1 MILE
3000	0	3000	6000 FEET
1	.5	0	1 KILOMETER

★15½

TRUE NORTH

MAGNETIC
NORTH
1982

183

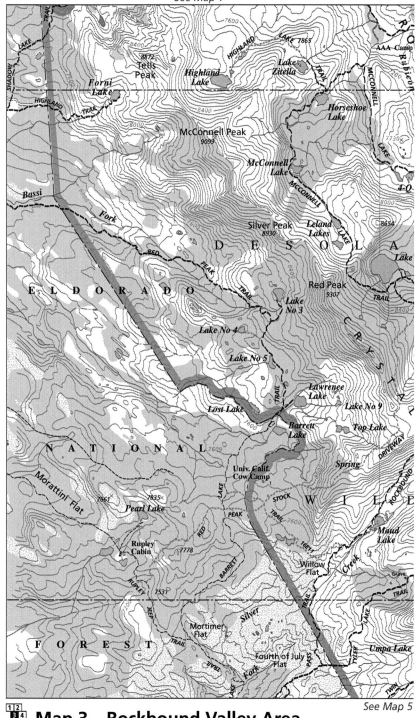

See Map 5

Map 3 – Rockbound Valley Area

See Map 4

185

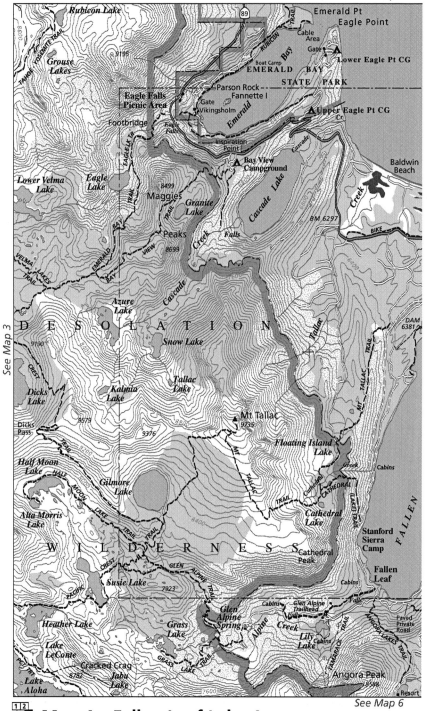

See Map 3

See Map 6

Map 4 – Fallen Leaf Lake Area

186

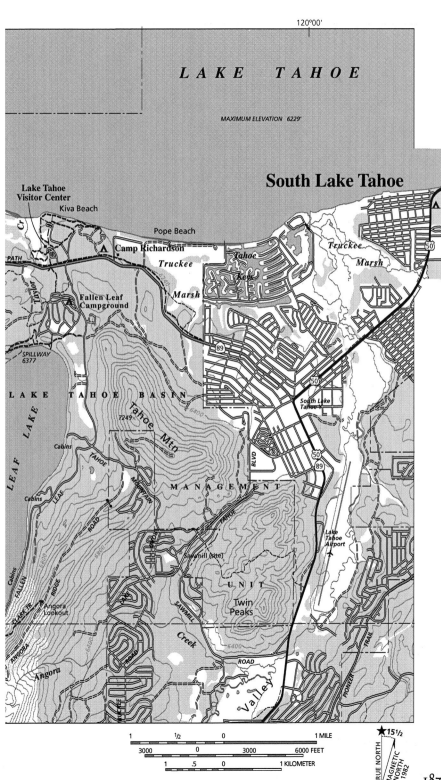

LAKE TAHOE

MAXIMUM ELEVATION 6229'

South Lake Tahoe

Lake Tahoe
Visitor Center
Kiva Beach

Pope Beach

PATH

Camp Richardson

Truckee

Tahoe
Keys

Truckee
Marsh

Fallen Leaf
Campground

Marsh

SPILLWAY
6377

LAKE   TAHOE   BASIN

Tahoe Mtn

7249'

Cabins

MANAGEMENT

Cabins

Lake
Tahoe
Airport

BLVD

South Lake
Tahoe

Sawmill (site)

UNIT

Twin
Peaks

Angora
Lookout

Creek

Angora

Valley

ROAD

1   1/2   0   1 MILE

3000   0   3000   6000 FEET

1   .5   0   1 KILOMETER

TRUE NORTH
MAGNETIC NORTH
1982
15½

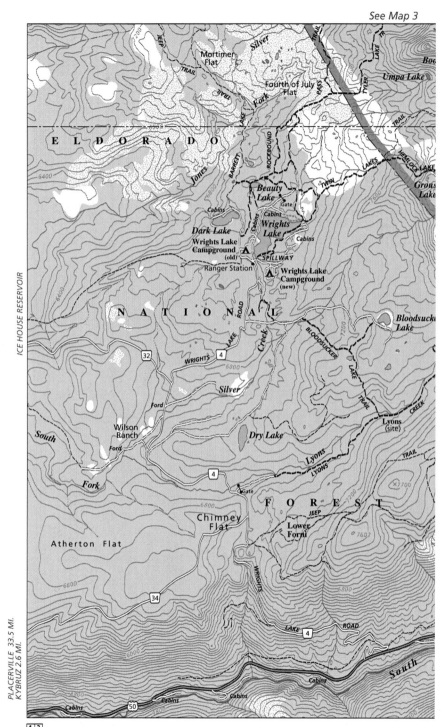

Map 5 – Wrights Lake Area

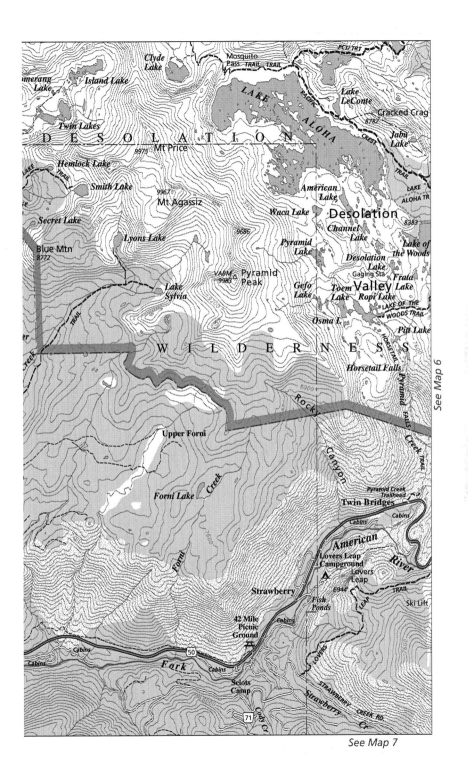

See Map 6

See Map 7

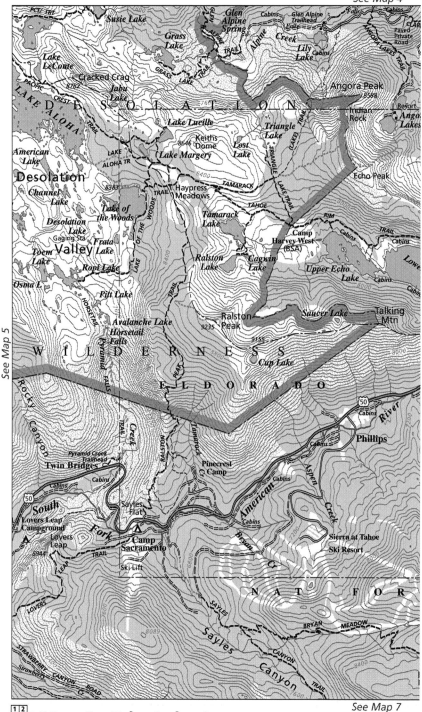

See Map 5

Map 6 – Echo Lake Area

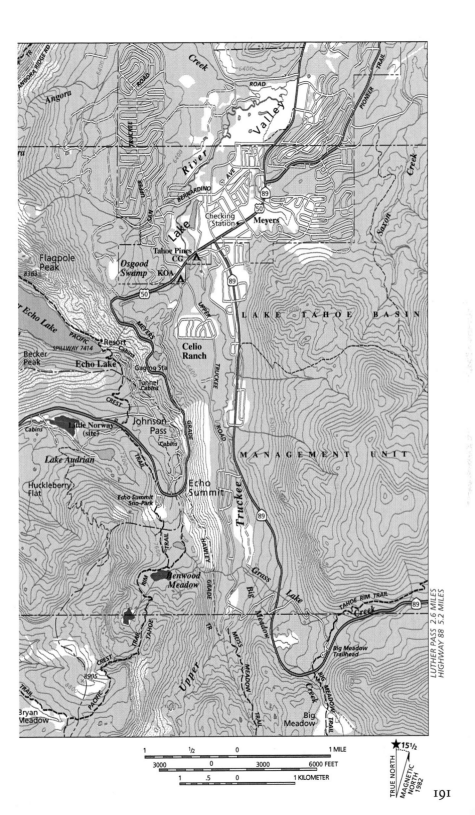

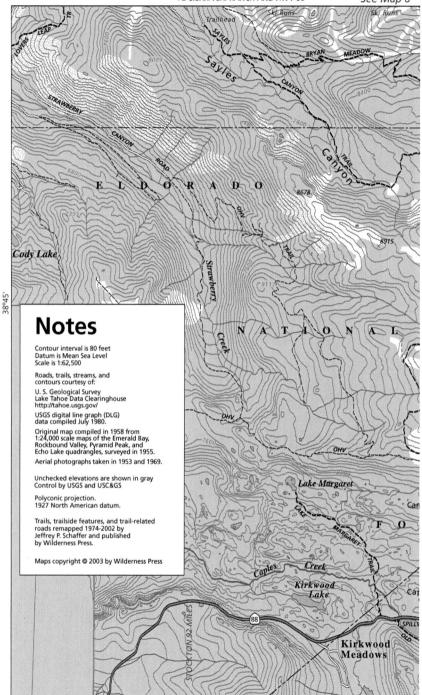

Notes

Contour interval is 80 feet
Datum is Mean Sea Level
Scale is 1:62,500

Roads, trails, streams, and
contours courtesy of:

U. S. Geological Survey
Lake Tahoe Data Clearinghouse
http://tahoe.usgs.gov/

USGS digital line graph (DLG)
data compiled July 1980.

Original map compiled in 1958 from
1:24,000 scale maps of the Emerald Bay,
Rockbound Valley, Pyramid Peak, and
Echo Lake quadrangles, surveyed in 1955.

Aerial photographs taken in 1953 and 1969.

Unchecked elevations are shown in gray
Control by USGS and USC&GS

Polyconic projection.
1927 North American datum.

Trails, trailside features, and trail-related
roads remapped 1974-2002 by
Jeffrey P. Schaffer and published
by Wilderness Press.

Maps copyright © 2003 by Wilderness Press

Map 7 – Upper Truckee River Area

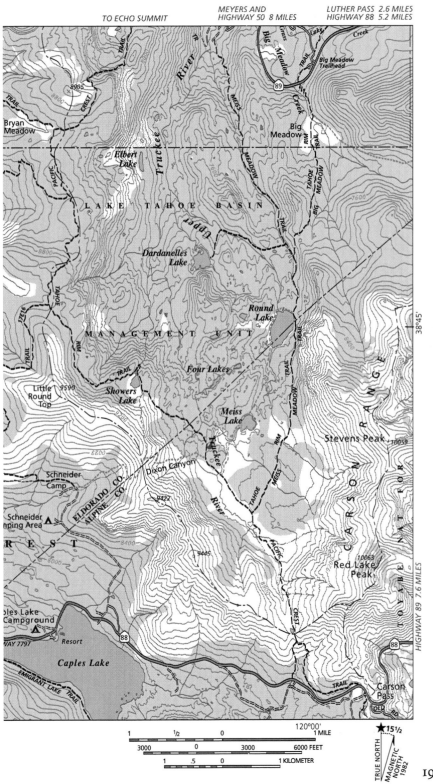

Big Meadow
Creek

Big Meadow
Trailhead

89

Bryan
Meadow

8905
8800

Elbert
Lake

Big
Meadow

L A K E   T A H O E   B A S I N

Dardanelles
Lake

Round
Lake

M A N A G E M E N T   U N I T

Four Lakes

Little
Round
Top

9590

Showers
Lake

Meiss
Lake

Stevens Peak
10059

Schneider
Camp

Dixon Canyon

9422

ELDORADO CO.
ALPINE CO.

Schneider
mping Area

R E S T

9445

Red Lake
Peak
10063

les Lake
Campground

Resort

88

C A R S O N   R A N G E

T O Y E B E   N A T   F O R

Caples Lake

EMIGRANT LAKE TRAIL

TRAIL

Carson
Pass

88

38°45'

HIGHWAY 89 7.6 MILES

120°00'

1   1/2   0   1 MILE

3000   0   3000   6000 FEET

1   .5   0   1 KILOMETER

TRUE NORTH
MAGNETIC
NORTH
1982

15½

193

Recommended Reading and Source Materials

General and Historical

Crippen, J. R., and B. R. Pavelka. 1970. *The Lake Tahoe Basin, California-Nevada*. U.S. Geological Survey Water-Supply Paper 1972, 56 p.

Farquhar, Francis P. 1965. *History of the Sierra Nevada*. Berkeley and Los Angeles: University of California Press, 262 p.

Reid, Robert L., ed. 1983. *A Treasury of the Sierra Nevada*. Berkeley: Wilderness Press, 363 p.

Scott, Edward B. 1957. *The Saga of Lake Tahoe*. Crystal Bay (Lake Tahoe), NV: Sierra-Tahoe Publishing Company, 519 p.

Hiking and Climbing

Carville, Mike. 1991. *Climber's Guide to Tahoe Rock*. Evergreen, CO: Chockstone Press, 295 p.

Darville, Fred T., Jr., M.D. 1998. *Mountaineering Medicine and Backcountry Medical Guide*. Berkeley: Wilderness Press, 110 p.

Hauserman, Tim. 2002. *The Tahoe Rim Trail: A Complete Guide for Hikers, Mountain Bikers, and Equestrians*. Berkeley: Wilderness Press, 252 p.

Schaffer, Jeffrey P. 2003. *Pacific Crest Trail: Northern California*. Berkeley: Wilderness Press, 360 p.

___. 2003. *The Tahoe Sierra*. Berkeley: Wilderness Press, 402 p.

Winnett, Thomas, with Melanie Findling. 1994. *Backpacking Basics*. Berkeley: Wilderness Press, 134 p.

Geology

Alley, Richard B. 2000. *The Two-Mile Time Machine: Ice Cores, Abrupt Climate Change, and Our Future*. Princeton, NJ: Princeton University Press, 229 p.

Bateman, Paul C., and Clyde Wahrhaftig. 1966. "Geology of the Sierra Nevada." In *Geology of Northern California* (Edgar H. Bailey, ed.). California Division of Mines and Geology

Bulletin 190, p. 107-169. (Best overview, but extremely dated.)

Curtis, Garniss H. 1954. "Mode of origin of pyroclastic debris in the Mehrten Formation of the Sierra Nevada." *University of California Publications in Geological Sciences*, v. 29, no. 9, p. 453-502.

Dodge, F.C.W., and P.V. Fillo. 1967. *Mineral Resources of the Desolation Primitive Area of the Sierra Nevada, California*. U.S. Geological Survey Bulletin 1261-A, 25 p.

Fisher, G. Reid. 1989. *Geologic map of the Mount Tallac roof pendant*. U.S. Geological Survey Map MF-1943.

___. 1990. "Middle Jurassic syntectonic conglomerate in the Mt. Tallac roof pendant, northern Sierra Nevada, California." In *Paleozoic and Early Mesozoic Paleogeographic Relations; Sierra Nevada, Klamath Mountains, and Related Terranes* (David S. Harwood and M. Meghan Miller, eds.). Geological Society of America Special Paper 255, p. 339-350.

Gardner, James V., Larry A. Mayer, and John E. Hughs Clarke. 2000. "Morphology and processes in Lake Tahoe (California-Nevada)." *Geological Society of America Bulletin*, v. 112, p. 736-46.

Graymer, Russell W., and David L. Jones. 1994. "Tectonic implications of radiolarian cherts from the Placerville Belt, Sierra Nevada Foothills, California: Nevadan-age continental growth by accretion of multiple terranes." *Geological Society of America Bulletin*, v. 106, p. 531-540.

House, Martha A., Brian P. Wernicke, and Kenneth A. Farley. 1998. "Dating topography of the Sierra Nevada, California, using apatite (U-Th)/He ages." *Nature*, v. 396, p. 66-69.

John, David A., and others. 1981. *Geologic Map of the Freel and Dardanelles Further Planning Areas, Alpine and El Dorado Counties, California*. U.S. Geological Survey Map MF-1322-A.

___. 1983. *Mineral Resource Potential Map of the Freel and Dardanelles Roadless Areas, Alpine and El Dorado Counties, California*. U.S. Geological Survey Map MF-1322-C.

Loomis, Alden A. 1983. *Geology of the Fallen Leaf Lake 15-Minute Quadrangle, El Dorado County, California*. California Division of Mines and Geology Map Sheet 32 (with 1981 24-p. text).

Schaffer, Jeffrey P. 1997. *The Geomorphic Evolution of the Yosemite Valley and Sierra Nevada Landscapes*. Berkeley: Wilderness Press, 388 p.

Slemmons, David B. 1966. "Cenozoic volcanism of the central Sierra Nevada, California." In *Geology of Northern California* (Edgar H. Bailey, ed.). California Division of Mines and Geology Bulletin 190, p. 199-208.

Biology

Carville, Julie Stauffer. 1989. *Hiking Tahoe's Wildflower Trails.* Edmonton, Alberta, Canada T6E 1X5: Lone Pine Publishing. 350 p.

Gaines, David. 1988. *Birds of Yosemite and the East Slope.* Lee Vining: Artemisia Press, 352 p.

Graf, Michael. 1999. *Plants of the Tahoe Basin.* Sacramento: California Native Plant Society Press, 308 p.

Grater, Russell K., and Tom A. Blaue. 1978. *Discovering Sierra Mammals.* El Portal: Yosemite Association, 174 p.

Hickman, James C., ed. 1993. *The Jepson Manual: Vascular Plants of California.* Berkeley and Los Angeles: University of California Press, 1400 p.

Horn, Elizabeth L. 1998. *Sierra Nevada Wildflowers.* Missoula, MT: Mountain Press, 215 p.

Jameson, E. W., Jr., and Hans J. Peeters. 1988. *California Mammals.* Berkeley and Los Angeles: University of California Press, 403 p.

Keator, Glenn. 1978. *Pacific Coast Berry Finder.* Berkeley: Nature Study Guild, 62 p.

Niehaus, Theodore P., and Charles L. Ripper. 1976. *A Field Guide to Pacific States Wildflowers.* Boston: Houghton Mifflin, 432 p.

Sibley, David Allen. 2000. *(National Audubon Society's) The Sibley Guide to Birds.* New York: Alfred A. Knopf, 544 p.

Stebbins, Robert C. 1998. *A Field Guide to Western Reptiles and Amphibians.* Boston: Houghton Mifflin, 360 p.

Storer, Tracy I., and Robert L. Usinger. 1989. *Sierra Nevada Natural History.* Berkeley and Los Angeles: University of California Press, 374 p.

Watts, Tom. 1973. *Pacific Coast Tree Finder.* Berkeley: Nature Study Guild, 62 p.

Weeden, Norman F. 1996. *A Sierra Nevada Flora.* Berkeley: Wilderness Press, 259 p.

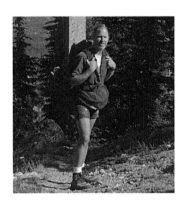

About the Author

Jeffrey P. Schaffer made his first backpacking trip in a 1962 traverse of the Grand Canyon, at age 19. The following year the climbing frenzy seized him, which lasted until about 1972, some 200 roped ascents later. In that year he began working on his first book for Wilderness Press, *The Pacific Crest Trail*. Between then and the late 1980s, he was the sole or principal author of 12 guidebooks, and had mapped about 4000 miles of trail for his books and 15-minute topographic maps. Innumerable observations while hiking made him seriously question conventional geological wisdom on the origin of mountain ranges, which led him to write a lengthly book on the origin of the Sierra Nevada landscapes, particularly Yosemite Valley. At the start of the millennium he was teaching geology and geography at Napa Valley College, introducing students to the Sierra Nevada and other lands.

Wilderness Press books authored or coauthored by Jeff include *Hiker's Guide to the High Sierra: Yosemite and Tuolumne Meadows, Pacific Crest Trail: Southern California, Pacific Crest Trail: Northern California, The Pacific Crest Trail, Vol. 2: Oregon and Washington, Lassen Volcanic National Park and Vicinity, Yosemite National Park, Desolation Wilderness and the South Lake Tahoe Basin, The Tahoe Sierra, Hiking the Big Sur Country: The Ventana Wilderness,* and *The Geomorphic Evolution of the Yosemite Valley and Sierra Nevada Landscapes.*

Index

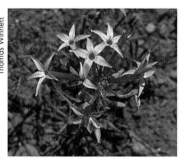

Ipomopsis aggregeta

Map Index

Desolation Wilderness

Desolation Wilderness